EBOLA

Edited by **Črtomir Podlipnik**

Ebola
http://dx.doi.org/10.5772/61360
Edited by Črtomir Podlipnik

Contributors
Yue Teng, Dan Feng, Zhe Xu, Jiangman Song, Xiaoping An, Colin Brown, Yan Yu, Yuan Jin, Alfonso Rodriguez-Morales, Jaime A. Cardona-Ospina, Alberto E. Paniz-Mondolfi, Sivia Fernanda-Urbano, Katherinn Melissa Nasner-Posso, Stefania Cruz-Calderón, Carlos E. Calvache-Benavides, Yudy Lorena Delgado-Pascuaza, Juan Camilo Castillo, Maria Yamile Alvarez-Ríos, Hamilton A. Marín-Rincón, Liceth Urrutia, Samuel Okware, Crtomir Podlipnik, Sebastian Pleško, Yassine Kasmi

Published by InTech
Janeza Trdine 9, 51000 Rijeka, Croatia

Publishing Process Manager Iva Lipovic
Technical Editor SPi Global
Cover InTech Design team

First published September, 2016
Printed in Croatia

Additional hard copies can be obtained from orders@intechopen.com

Ebola, Edited by Črtomir Podlipnik
p. cm.
Print ISBN 978-953-51-2517-4
Online ISBN 978-953-51-2518-1

For EU product safety concerns:
IN TECH d.o.o., Prolaz Marije Krucifikse Kozulić 3, 51000 Rijeka, Croatia,
info@intechopen.com or visit our website at intechopen.com.

Meet the editor

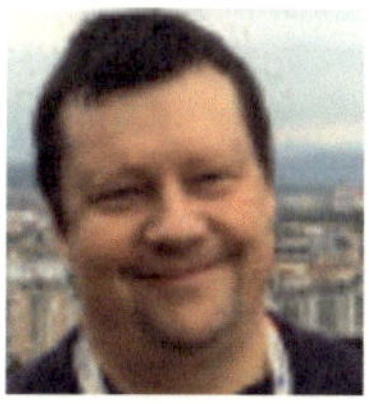

Dr. Črtomir Podlipnik obtaineded his PhD in the field of theoretical chemistry at the University of Ljubljana, Slovenia, under the supervision of Prof. Jože Koller. Afterwards, he joined the group of Prof. Anna Bernardi (University of Milan, Italy), where he was involved in the designing of cholera toxin inhibitors. Currently, he is working as an assistant professor at the Faculty of Chemistry and Chemical Technology, University of Ljubljana, Slovenia. He has great scientific interest in the research of relevant biomolecular systems, and with his valuable comprehensive knowledge in this field, he actively participates in many projects, including research of Ebola.

Contents

Preface

The recent outbreak of the Ebola virus disease (EVD) in West Africa reminded us that an effective antiviral treatment still does not exist, despite the significant progress that has recently been made in understanding the biology and pathology of this lethal disease. Aside from the overwhelming health effects, the Ebola epidemic also influenced the social and economic situations in Liberia, Guinea, and Sierra Leone. Projections from the World Bank have shown long-term damage that exceed $2.2 billion for the year of 2015, which represents more than 10% in the gross domestic product (GDP) of these three countries.

The book *Ebola* is an up-to-date resource of know-how about various aspects of the Ebola virus (EBOV) and the related disease. Many experts from different fields of science and from different parts of the world contributed to the creation of this book.

The first section of the book describes epidemiology. In this section, the reader may find the interesting contribution about the firsthand experience in managing Ebola in low-resource settings, with a detailed description of the Sudan Ebola virus and the Bundibugyo Ebola virus outbreaks occurred in Uganda from 2000 to 2012. The Uganda experience is extremely valuable and provides opportunities for further research of described strategies that could improve the management and control of Ebola in low-resource countries. In the next chapter, authors have revisited the various stages of the EVD outbreak, from early triage and case definitions, through ramping up isolation and treatment capacity, to how best to retain and develop resilience in health systems, alongside research efforts and outbreak control principles. They have highlighted that collaborations and partnerships at national and international levels are vital in building health systems for early surveillance and management of emerging infections. In the last chapter of this section, the reader may read about the experience of preparedness as well as risk assessment done in Latin America regarding the threat of Ebola for this region.

The second section of the book is dedicated to genetic analysis of the Ebola virus. This section includes a very interesting study of the genomic portrait of haplotype diversity in EBOV from the 1976 to the 2014 outbreaks. The authors of this study detected the diversity of viral haplotypes with systematic calculation of phylogeographic distribution in EBOV. Their observations highlight how variations of the Ebola virus are substantially different in virulence or transmissibility in comparison to the virus lineages associated with 2014 outbreaks in Sierra Leone, which provides a clue to understand the 2014 EBOV spreading. The second chapter of Teng et al. offers a systematic investigation of microRNA-like small RNAs in EBOV genome by bioinformatics tools. Their findings may shed light on the underlying molecular mechanisms of the pathological process of Ebola virus disease (EVD).

The last section of the book is dedicated to the structure and pathogenesis of the Ebola virus, which is recognized as one of the most "intelligent" viruses, with mysterious simplicity in its genome, which encodes only seven genes. Despite of its genetic simplicity, the virus has complex and very deadly lifestyle. The first targets of Ebola virus are typically immune cells, such as dendritic cells and macrophages whose primary function is to alert the immune system to the incoming threat. When it damages early immune cells, Ebola becomes very efficient in its devastating action. As the dendritic cells and macrophages fall apart, they produce a cytokine storm, which further harms immune cells and also other tissues. Ebola then attacks many other organs. Unlike HIV, Ebola is able to invade almost all other human cells, except for lymphocytes. The knowledge about EBOV structure and pathogenesis, collected in the book, may contribute in the task of searching an effective medication against Ebola.

In the first instance, the editor of this book would like to thank the authors for their contributions; many thanks go to the great support of personnel from the InTech publisher, especially to Mrs. Ivona Lovrić, who carried up the Ebola book project. Many thanks go also to my close collaborator Mr. Sebastian Pleško, for his continued and valuable assistance in this project. The editor of this book is also grateful for the support of the Slovenian Research Agency through the research program P1-0201.

Črtomir Podlipnik

Faculty of Chemistry and Chemical Technology,

University of Ljubljana,

Ljubljana, Slovenia

Section 1

Epidemiology of Ebola Viral Disease

Chapter 1

Managing Ebola in Low-resource Settings: Experiences from Uganda

Samuel Okware

Additional information is available at the end of the chapter

http://dx.doi.org/10.5772/63056

Abstract

Five outbreaks of Ebola virus disease of the Sudan Ebola virus and the Bundibugyo Ebola virus occurred in Uganda from 2000 to 2012. The attack rates and the case fatality rates were much higher for the former than the later. Fever and bleeding manifestations associated with the clustering of cases were typical clinical features. Close contact with infected person was probably the major route of spread. Apparent asymptomatic and atypical Ebola infection was demonstrated in some close contacts, suggesting past unrecognised exposure or cross-reacting antibodies. A zoonotic connection was apparent in monkeys and asymptomatic villagers. The Ministry of Health together with its partners contained the outbreaks, sometimes with delays, but at least once promptly. Early detection and communication yielded the best ideal outcomes. A community-based response ensured timely case search and contact tracing for the isolation and management of patients. The syndrome-based EVD case definition and the laboratory screening tests for Ebola were used to detect cases. However, their unknown specificity and sensitivity and their low positive predictive values were a major weakness in the screening process. Validation of the criteria and the tests at the local level was essential. There were gaps in isolation procedures as 64% of the health care workers were infected after the isolation units were established. Palliative treatment was an important part of management as it improved survival and public confidence. Therefore, survival and not just quarantine must be emphasized and be a critical component of EVD management. Substantial investment in human resource for health is needed to attract, reward, retain and compensate health workers. Collaboration and partnerships at national and international level is vital in building health systems for early surveillance and management of emerging infections. The Uganda experience provides opportunities for further research on some of these strategies that could improve the management and control of Ebola in low resource countries.

Keywords: Ebola, outbreaks, detection, management, resources

1. Introduction

1.1. Ebola Virus Disease (EVD)

Five outbreaks of EVD occurred in Uganda between 2000 and 2012 [1–4]. In this paper, we describe our experience, challenges and opportunities that existed during the Ebola outbreaks in Uganda. The Gulu outbreak in 2000 was the largest and most complex occurrence in the midst of an insurgency and severely deteriorated social services [5]. The first reported outbreak of EVD was identified in 1976, in the DR Congo, on the border of Sudan [6]. Since then, there have been 26 outbreaks in Equatorial Africa occurring in DR Congo, Gabon, Sudan and Uganda. The majority of these outbreaks were minor. The most serious outbreak occurred in West Africa in 2014 causing some 23,000 cases and 11,000 deaths in Liberia, Guinea and Sierra Leone [7]. Of the five known species (EBOV, SUDV, RESTV, TAFV, BDBV) only three are associated with disease. The *Zaire ebolavirus* has the highest case fatality (90%) while the *Sudan ebolavirus* is medium at 50–55% [8]. The *case fatality for the Bundibugyo ebolavirus* is low at 34%. There is no known cure yet for the disease. Ebola symptoms mimic several common diseases in the tropics including malaria.

Lymphoid tissue such as the liver, spleen, and thymus are critical targets which are often severely damaged leading to liver necrosis, bleeding manifestations and shock. Organ damage leads to a series of metabolic dysfunctions which maintain blood pressure homeostasis [9, 10]. Fruit bats are potential reservoirs of the *Zaire ebolavirus* through direct contact with freshly killed bats or when ingested as food [11]. Asymptomatic infection of between 4– 15% among the pygmies in Gabon and DR Congo [12] has been demonstrated suggesting some previous exposure to Ebola or cross-reacting strains Ebola has been isolated from seminal fluids 61 days after onset of illness [13]. This may be a potential source of infection in large outbreaks in low resource settings. Direct contact with body fluids of an infected person (dead or alive) via broken skin or mucosal surfaces is probably the most important route of infection [14]. The intramuscular route is perceived to be more effective [14]. In poor healthcare settings, contaminated needles and syringes are likely sources of infection. Re-use of needles, for instance, played a key role in escalating the epidemics in Sudan and DR Congo in 1976 [15].

1.2. Ebola outbreaks in Uganda 2000–2012

In 2000, some 425 cases and 224 deaths occurred in Gulu district and 31 health care workers were infected. The affected village was Rwot Obillo, 14 km north of Gulu towards the border with South Sudan. The local community was inaccessible because of on-going military operations against insurgency in the area. On the 8th of October, 2000, three student nurses died in Lacor hospital [1]. On the 12th of October the Sudan Ebola virus was confirmed among the blood samples taken. Nearly 2 million people most of whom lived in camps were at risk in the region [16]. Rural residents commuted to Gulu town for fear of Ebola and abduction from LRA rebels. Two patients in Gulu escaped to Masindi and Mbarara districts, but were followed, isolated and contained. The outbreak lasted 6 months.

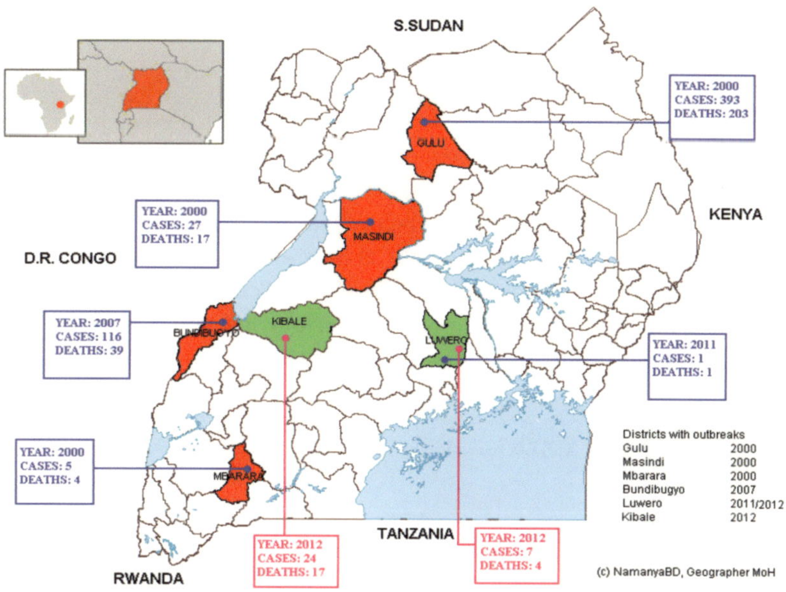

Figure 1. Outbreaks of Ebola in Uganda by district, 2000–2012. Source: Adapted from Ebola outbreak reports 2000-2012; WHO Health Mapper Mapping software, version 4.2

Four more Ebola outbreaks caused by Sudan Ebola virus occurred with increasing frequency in 2011 and 2012 [3, 4]. The primary cases were from rural areas. In 2007, the Bundibugyo Ebola virus caused the second outbreak [17]. Major transmission of the early cases was associated with patient care and burial rituals [2]. The diagnosis was delayed but once detected it took just 3 weeks to contain the outbreak [18]. Serious action was launched and isolation established. Community mobilisation and action contained the outbreak. Some 116 cases and 39 deaths were confirmed, and 14 health care workers were among the victims. Unlike in the Gulu outbreak, the health care workers contracted infection before the isolation units were established.

1.2.1. Luwero outbreaks: 2011, 2012

More outbreaks occurred in Luwero in 2011 and 2012. Early detection was key in limiting the Luwero 2011 outbreak to a single case [3]. On the 5th of May, a 13-year-old girl was admitted to Bombo hospital with a history of fever, diarrhea and vomiting. She was isolated and her blood was investigated. She developed vaginal bleeding and deteriorated and died the following day. The Sudan Ebola subtype was detected and confirmed. The results were communicated quickly to the community on the media and by house to house messages by word of mouth. Contacts were followed up by the community. No new case was discovered or reported. This is the ideal desirable scenario for Ebola containment. In December 2012, hardly six months after the Kibaale outbreak, a second Ebola outbreak resurfaced in Luwero district [4]. The outbreak was confirmed within days and contained in 6 weeks leaving 7 cases with 4 deaths.

1.2.2. Kibaale outbreak, 2012

Earlier in July 2012, an Ebola outbreak occurred in the district of Kibaale [4]. The index case was a 16-year-old female from a remote rural community. She fell sick while preparing forest land with her husband for planting season. On admission, she complained of fever, diarrhea and vomiting. She developed a nose bleed just before she died. Nine relatives who participated at the funeral died including a mother, and several sisters who contracted the infection died. A priest who led the burial ceremony also died. One health care worker who attended to her also died. Community action followed up 408 contacts during which some 24 cases and 17 deaths were confirmed. The outbreak was contained in six weeks.

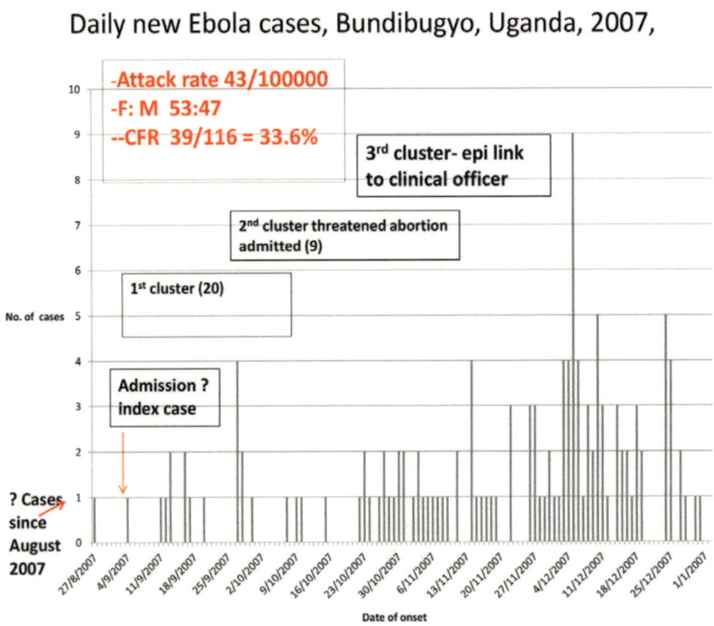

Figure 2. Clustering of Ebola cases by week, Bundibugyo, 2007–2008.

1.3. Clinical manifestations of cases

Cases were identified using an adapted WHO syndrome based criteria for "suspect", "probable" and "confirmed" cases. Clustering of cases (**Figure 2**) associated with sudden onset of fever particularly among health care givers is highly suspicious. The most common symptoms were fever, headache, anorexia and diarrhea. However, in a few cases (15%) no fever was observed in patients on admission. This observation and unsuspected source of infection poses [5] a potential danger to health care givers. Bleeding tendencies occurred in about 50% of the cases of SUDV, but less than 30% in the BDBGV outbreaks. The diagnosis was often complicated by the several locally endemic febrile conditions which mimicked Ebola such as malaria which accounts for up to 50% of cases at the outpatient clinics Uganda.

1.4. Risk factors

Some significant observations were made on risk factors. The outbreaks occurred between June and December coinciding with the rainy season, during which fields are prepared for planting. It was also a fruit season. Known primary cases occurred in the rural areas. Access to fruits partially eaten by non-human primates was common during the season and may have been a potential source of infection.

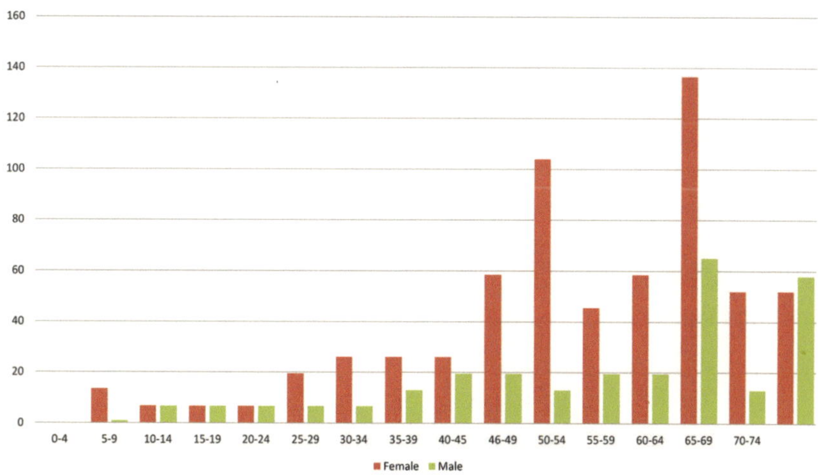

Figure 3. Attack rates per 10,000 inhabitants by gender and age, Gulu district, Uganda, 2000.

Age and gender were associated with infection in Gulu district. There was a 16-fold risk increase with increasing age between children and the elderly and was highest at 60–64 years age group. The attack rates among children between 5–14 years were the lowest (**Figure 3**). In Gulu district, the high risk in elderly women is associated with their role in cleansing and preparing the dead before burial [19]. In Bundibugyo too, participation in some ritual ceremonies was associated with a 7-fold increase in risk [2]. Contact with a known case carried between four to sevenfold increases in risk. Visiting a hospital or a hospitalized patient was associated with a ninefold increase in risk. The possibility of a zoonotic connection or cross reacting local strains was observed as some SUDV Ig G antibodies were confirmed in the monkey carcasses and a few asymptomatic local residents [1].

Year	District	Cases detected	Deaths	CFR
2000	Gulu	393	203	51.7%
	Mbarara	5	4	80.0%
	Masindi	27	17	63.0%

Year	District	Cases detected	Deaths	CFR
Total[a]		**425**[b]	**224**	**52.7%**
2007	Bundibugyo	116[c]	39	34 %
2011	Luwero	1	1	100%
2012, Jun-Aug	Kibaale	24[d]	17	70%
2012, Nov-Dec	Luwero	7	4	57%

Source: Ebola situation analysis reports 2000-2012

Table 1. Ebola cases by year and district, Uganda, 2000–2012

2. The national response

The national response was multisectoral and led by the President who directed all sectors to get mobilised and participate. The Ebola national task force in the Ministry of Health led the implementation of the strategic work plans. The task force reported to the Office of the Prime Minister, the leader of government business. Working groups were set up in the following areas: planning and coordination, surveillance and laboratory service, public education, case management, and logistics management (**Figure 4**).

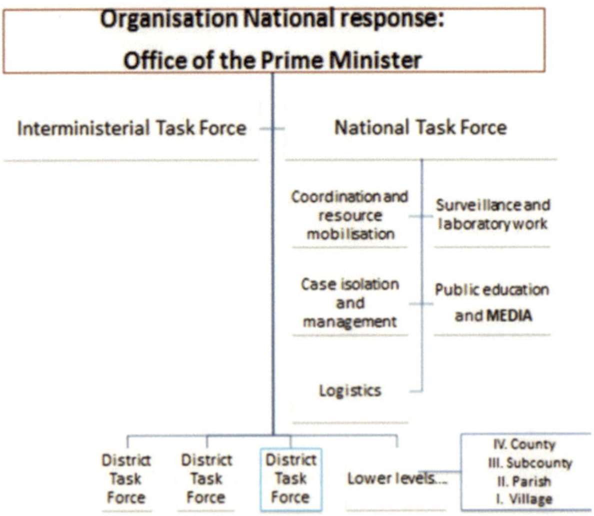

Figure 4. Organization of the national response.

One national joint plan was developed to which the various collaborators subscribed both at national and international level. International support including expertise was integrated into the national plan endorsed by national and international stakeholders including bilateral development partners.

A syndrome-based case definition was adapted from the WHO[1] guidelines and used for community-based active case search. A flow chart (**Figure 5**) integrated and harmonized the participation of the various actors. Community mobilization focused on public education and active case search by the community optimized through media. Full participation of church leaders, school principals and local political leadership and mobile teams was the cornerstone of community effort. Isolation and triage units were set up in district hospitals. Health care workers were recruited and paid risk allowances to boost motivation and dedication. Workers with previous experience and institutional memory were preferred and redeployed. Daily report updates and press briefings were openly communicated to the public at all levels. Similar arrangements were set up at the district, county, sub county, parish and village levels (**Figure 4**).

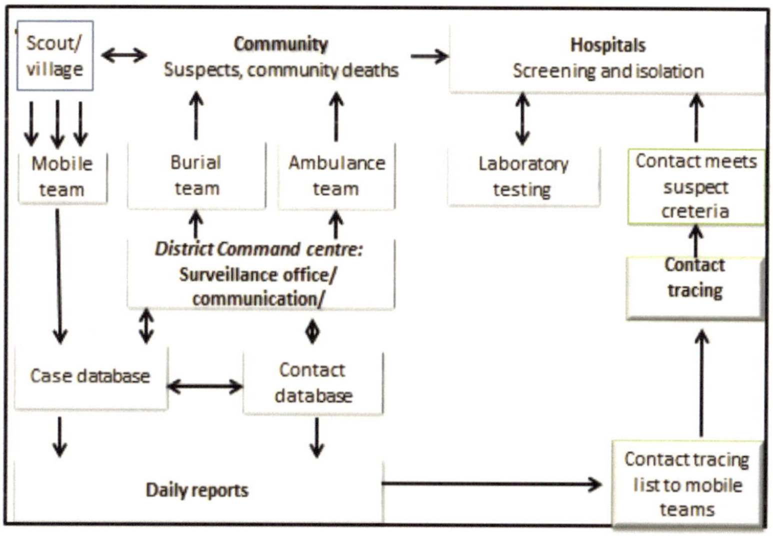

Figure 5. Flow chart for community based surveillance.

A cascade of training starting with training of trainers countrywide was carried out within days. Each village appointed a village health team led by a chairman and secretary (scout) to coordinate the implementation. At district level, a district task force coordinated the response. Incentives were paid to them for each Ebola case reported and revalidated. Burial and safe disposal of the dead was coordinated by a district burial coordinator who liaised with the hospital coordinator and the village health teams. Trained burial teams with past experience were recruited, retrained and liaised with the village scout to ensure safe and timely burials. On discharge, the patients went through a series of stringent protocols and check lists conducted by trained counsellors. Post Ebola clinics and clubs were set up for follow up of health and social outcomes.

---

1 Adapted from the WHO (2003)

3. Examples of best practice

3.1 Successful community action

There were some examples when timely community action effectively stopped the spread of these Ebola outbreaks. The best examples were demonstrated in Masindi district (2000) and the Luwero district (2011). A known case escaped from Gulu hospital to her ancestral home in Masindi district because her nurse died. The patient belonged to an extended family of 73 members residing in the district. The local community imposed quarantine on the members of the extended family. Transmission was prevented beyond the extended family - of the 27 new cases in the district 25 were from the extended family and only one case came from the general population (**Figure 6**). Thus, transmission beyond the extended family of the index case was effectively prevented by early detection and action and quarantine imposed by the community [20].

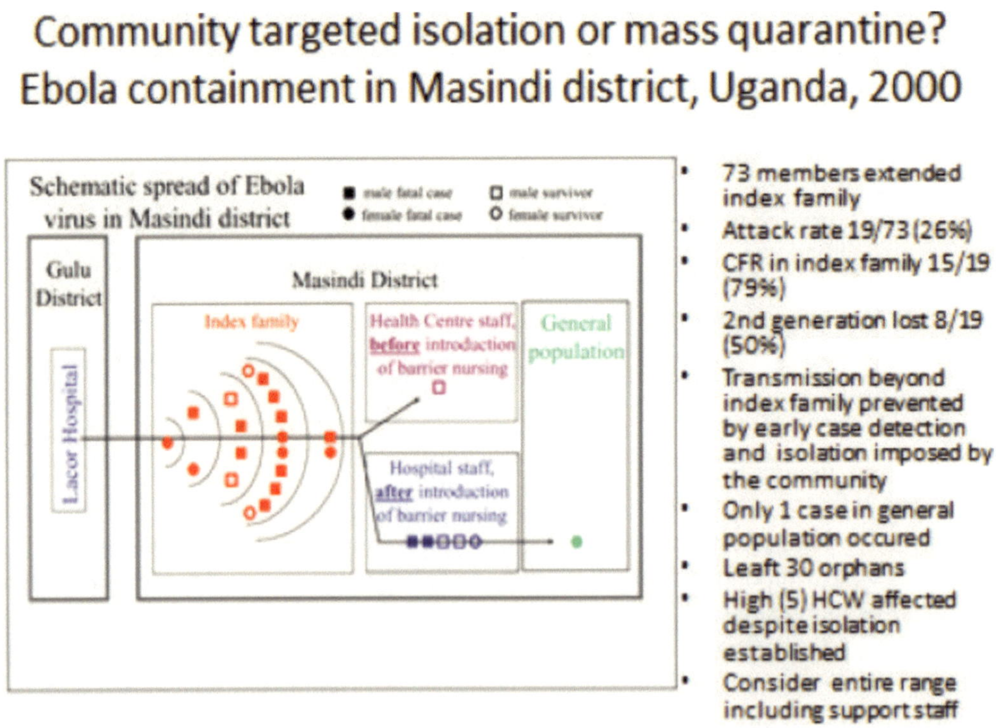

Figure 6. Community based Ebola containment of Ebola in Masindi district, Uganda, 2000.

3.2 Early detection and action

The Luwero outbreak of 2011 demonstrated the critical role of early detection and action in containing the outbreaks [3]. The single case outbreak was contained within one week. This excellent outcome occurred when a case was promptly diagnosed and confirmed to have Ebola. She was immediately isolated and the community was mobilized to start the public response including education, active contact tracing and isolation. This is the most desirable outcome as demonstrated by the critical timelines in **Figure 7**. The need for early diagnosis and action cannot be overemphasized.

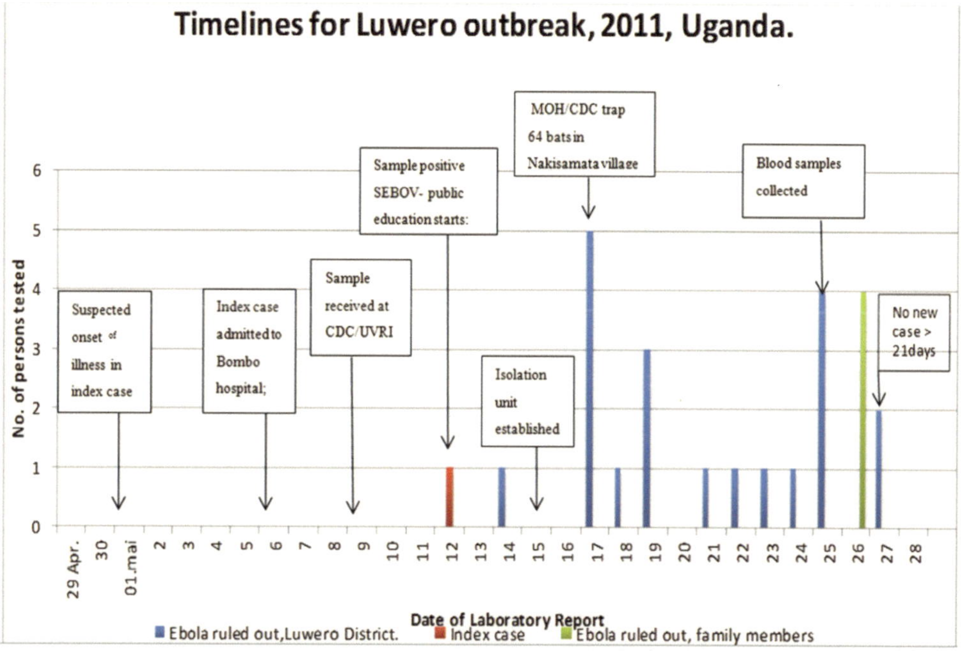

Figure 7. Early Ebola detection and containment, Luwero district, Uganda, 2011.

4. Challenges

4.1 Delayed action

Delays in early detection prolonged the spread of infection and late action. The respective districts experienced the following delays: in the districts of Gulu district (6 weeks delay); Bundibugyo (6 months); Kibaale (6 weeks). Most (75%) of the delays were at community level. Once the diagnosis was made, it took between 5 and 17 days to contain the outbreaks in Luwero and Kibaale respectively: only 5 days in Luwero; some 17 days in Kibaale. The corresponding figure for the Gulu epidemic was longer (91 days). It also took 41 days to contain the Bundibugyo outbreak. Thus late detection facilitated the extensive spread of the infection in both instances.

District	Gulu, 2007		Bundibugyo, 2007		Kibaale, 2012		Luwero, 2012	
Time	Date	Days since onset	Date	Days since onset	Date	Days since onset	Date	Days since onset
Onset of strange disease in community	19/09/2000	0	07/08/2007	0	12/6/2012	0	13/10/12	0
Report to Ministry Health	9/10/2000	20	27/09//2007	51	12/07/2012	30	7/11/2012	24
Investigation: Blood sampled	12/10/2000	23	29/09/2007	53	13/07/2012	31	8/11/2012	25
Blood confirmation Ebola	14/10/2000	25	28/11/2007	60	27/07/2012	45	12/11/2012	29
Declaration national action	15/10/2000	26	29/11/2007	61	28/07/2012	46	13/11/2012	30
Last case	14/01/2001	91	08/01/2008	71	14/08/2012	63	17/11/2012	34
Total days epidemic lasted		**117**		**101**		**63**		**34**
From laboratory confirmation to last case		91		41		17		5

Source: Ebola situation analysis reports 2000-2012

Table 2. Timelines from onset of illness to containment by district, Uganda, 2000–2012.

District	Identified by mobile teams	Revalidated by supervisors as cases	Regarded by supervisors as non-cases	Positive predictive value (%)
Gulu	1069	536	533	50.1
Bundibugyo	192	116	76	60.4
Kibaale	115	24	91	20.8
Luwero	36	7	29	19.4

*. Reclassified later to 425 cases only.

Table 3. Positive predictive value by case definition by district, Uganda.

4.2 Validity of case definition

There were weaknesses in the application of the clinical syndrome case definition. The sensitivity and specificity of the definition were not known. The positive predictive value of the criteria used was low (Table 3). Some atypical Ebola cases presented without fever or bleeding. Fever was absent in 15% of cases while bleeding tendencies were observed only in 30-53% of admissions in Gulu. The validity of the case definition too was not known at local level. The positive predictive value of the case definition was low. Reassessment by supervisors validated less than half as true cases. Table 3 shows the low positive predictive values in the districts of Luwero (19.4%), Kibaale (20.8%), Bundibugyo (60.4%) and Gulu (50.1%).

4.3 Laboratory -challenges in reliability

Laboratory tests helped in the management of admissions and their discharge. Simple tests were used to detect and confirm Ebola: PCR, antigen detection, and immunoglobulin 1g M, and very rarely virus isolation. Surprisingly, less than 50% of the "suspected" and "probable" cases yielded positive laboratory results. Only half of the suspected and probable cases yielded positive laboratory results (Table 4). This low positive predictive value for the laboratory tests is a major weakness and delayed early diagnosis and action. The sensitivity and specificity and positive predictive values of the tests were also not known. The local validation of these tests is therefore essential. It is therefore critical to build laboratory capacity and skills at the national level to support outbreak management as well as conduct serosurveys in the population.

Laboratory status	Number	Proportion %
Gulu district		
Laboratory positive	195	45.8
Bundibugyo district		
Laboratory positive	42	21.9
Laboratory negative	74	38.5
Laboratory negative but probable	76	39.6
Total tested	**192**	**100**
Total lab positive and probable combined (42+76)/192	116	60.4

Table 4. Proportion of positive laboratory results of suspected Ebola cases by district, 2000–2012.

5 Case management: challenges and opportunities

5.1 Infection control and barrier nursing

Despite availability of personal protective materials, gaps remained in the practice of barrier nursing. These gaps were more pronounced among support staff especially drivers, cleaners and attendants. In Gulu, nosocomial infection persisted as 64% of the 31 health care workers got infected after the measures were put in place. Of the 6 health care workers infected in Masindi, five got infected after barrier nursing was instituted. In contrast, the infections among staff occurred before isolation units were established in Bundibugyo. Overcrowding and inadequate staff and supplies was a common feature in the isolation wards. Proper and timely use of protective materials was sometimes not followed especially when the patients were relatives. Procedures for washing and cleansing of ambulances were often taken lightly as gadgets such as cell phones were sometimes used indiscriminately. There was complacency in the general wards. A false sense of security could have been created by establishment of isolation units hence the need to train all workers in infection control. The surgical and maternity wards in particular were a major source of new inadvertent infections. Regular drills and training are essential within healthcare settings. It must also be extended to all other support staff including administrators, drivers and relatives providing bed side nursing.

5.2 Human resource and financing challenges

Caring for Ebola is a labor intensive and costly undertaking. For instance, the estimated direct costs of treating an Ebola case in the most affected countries in West Africa (Guinea, Sierra Leone and Liberia) ranged from USD 500 to 900 for those surviving and much more for the non survivors [21]. In the USA the costs of caring for one such patient was about USD 350,000 per week [22]. In Uganda, the government budget allocation for the health sector is USD 28 per capita. Therefore external support was mobilized and funds had to be diverted from the primary health care programmes in order to mount the national response. Human resources for health too are a major constraint in health delivery in Africa. Unlike developed countries, Uganda has a doctor: population ratio of 1:25,000 and the corresponding figure for nurses is 1:4000. Low salaries and lack of motivation continue to undermine performance. Poor motivation and low salaries did not attract health care workers into the isolation units leave alone the health facility. Risk allowances were introduced and this incentive provided the much needed motivation and improved performance in the isolation units. The availability of personal protective materials maintained staff confidence and commitment in the isolation wards. This demonstrated that the workers if adequately compensated can improve performance. Thus workers when well-paid and motivated can perform beyond expectations. Compensation was provided for the health care workers who died in the line of duty, but not for the other non-medical victims. A social health insurance scheme should be considered for future outbreaks.

5.3 Improving Survivalsurvival

Differences in severity and survival were demonstrated between the two Ebola subtypes. Unlike in the Gulu outbreak, the later did not spread to other districts. The attack rates and the case fatality rates were higher in Sudan subtype (Table 5). The case fatality rate was higher (53.1%), in the Gulu outbreak compared with that in Bundibugyo (34%). The attack rates were also lower for the Bundibugyo virus than that in Gulu, p=0.001. However, the observed outcomes in severity and survival may also have been associated to differences on condition on admission, bleeding manifestation, and possible antigenic differences. It was also observed that death was more associated with bleeding tendencies and vomiting, p= < 0.001. The long term effects on survivors showed increased risk of chronic health outcomes after recovery. Of the 70 survivors followed for 2 years in Bundibugyo, 14% had blurred vision, 28% had retro-orbital pain, and 23% had hearing loss. Difficulty in swallowing, muscle pain and memory loss was also reported [23]. Also, the Gulu Ebola survivors were unable to resume work one year post recovery [24].

Parameter	Ebola cases by case definition		
	Gulu, n= 324 p=value	Bundibugyo, n=116	
% Male cases (95% CI)	37 (32.0–42.4)	53 (43.5–61.7)	0.005
% Women cases (95% CI)	63 (57.7–68.2)	47 (38.3–56.5)	0.005
Attack rates/100,000 population (95% CI)	97(79–118) 0.001	43 (31–58)	
Case fatality rate % (95% CI)	53.1 (47.7–58.5)	34 (25.0–42.2)	0.005

Table 5. Attack rates and case fatality by district, 2000–2007.

Isolation isolated cases, provided quality care, improved survival and increased public trust. Patient survival differed from outbreak to outbreak but improved as management of palliative care was established. In Gulu, survival improved over time (**Figure 8**). Mortality declined from 100% at the onset, to just around 10% towards the end of the outbreak. Timely community detection promoted care and survival. Motivation of care givers was critical to this improved performance of health care workers. It was demonstrated that quality palliative care positively influenced survival [1]. Future interventions therefore should integrate health staff motivation in their budgets.

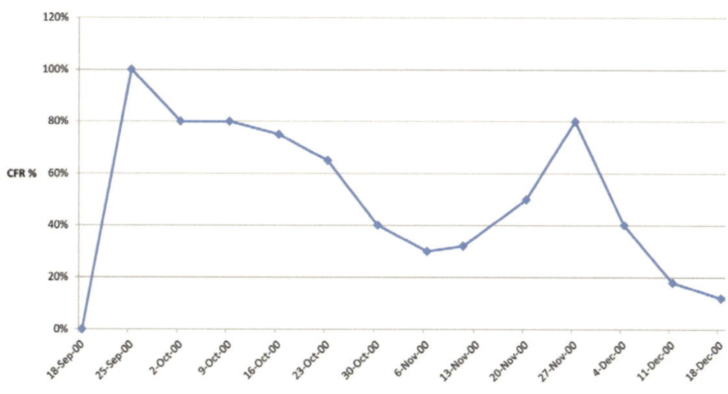

Figure 8. Case fatality rate of Ebola cases by week, Gulu district, Uganda, 2000.

6. Conclusion

Early detection and action resulted in the best outcomes for the outbreak containment. Community leadership and mobilization, including the media for action was vital in managing these Ebola outbreaks. The need to strengthen laboratory capacity for early detection of the infection cannot be overemphasized. Supportive treatment improved lives, reduced case fatality, isolated cases and indeed increased public confidence and health seeking behavior. Care and survival and not just quarantine should therefore be emphasized as a critical component of the interventions. There were serious gaps in barrier nursing as nosocomial infections continued despite institution of isolation units. Infection control strategies should be institutionalized to protect both the health workers and the support staff in the units and the general wards. There is a need to develop and implement a human resource strategy and plan that attracts rewards and retains health workers. Such plans should strengthen health care systems in order to respond effectively to future epidemics. There is a need for the international partnerships and collaboration to be strengthened so as to augment the national efforts. Such partnerships should build capacity for health systems for surveillance and care.

Surveillance of emerging infections should be strengthened by establishing networks and centers of excellence for sharing of information and monitoring emerging infections. Inventories and rapid response teams at national and international level should be shared so as to provide timely emergency stocks, expertise and technical support. The large outbreaks especially in West Africa impacted badly on social services and the economy. Early detection and action based on community effort remains the best option for low resource settings, which capacity should be integrated into primary health care and village health teams to mitigate post Ebola health outcomes.

Appendices

APPENDIX 1
Adapted WHO *Case definition of Ebola virus disease for Uganda*

Suspected cases	• Sudden onset of *fever and at least 4 of the following* symptoms in a resident of or visitor to the affected areas in the district: *vomiting, diarrhea, abdominal pain, conjunctivitis, skin rash, unexplained bleeding from any body part, muscle pain, intense fatigue, difficulty swallowing, difficulty breathing, hiccups, or headache* since suspected onset, • OR sudden *onset of fever* in any person who had *contact* with a person with *suspected, probable, or confirmed* EHF • OR *sudden death* in a person in the community without any other explanation.
Probable case	• *Suspected* EHF in any person (dead or alive) with *at least* 3 of the following symptoms: *vomiting, diarrhoea, or unexplained bleeding from any site, conjunctivitis, or skin rash;* AND

	• Either an epidemiologic *link* to a person with probable or confirmed EHF, OR • Either no specimen collected for laboratory testing or a negative laboratory result in a specimen collected 0-3 days after onset of symptoms in a person with suspected EHF.
Confirmed case	• Laboratory confirmation of infection by isolation of virus from any body fluid or tissue, OR • Detection *of viral antigen* in any body fluid or tissue by antigen-detection ELISA, reverse transcription-PCR, or immuno-histochemistry, OR • Demonstration of serum Ebola virus-specific IgG antibodies by ELISA, with or without IgM, in any person with suspected or probable EHF.
Contact	A person who had slept in the same household and/or had direct physical contact with a person (dead or alive) with suspected, probable, or confirmed EHF, and/or had been exposed to an infected person or to an infected person's secretions, excretions, tissues, or linen within 3 weeks after that person's onset of illness.

Author details

Samuel Okware

Address all correspondence to: okwares@gmail.com

Director General, Uganda National Health Research Organisation, Entebbe, Uganda

REFERENCES

[1] Okware S.I., *Three Ebola outbreaks in Uganda 2000-2011, in Center for International Health, Bergen, School of Medicine* 2015, University of Bergen, Bergen Norway.

[2] Wamala J.F., et al., *Ebola hemorrhagic fever associated with novel virus strain, Uganda, 2007-2008. Emerging infectious diseases, 2010.* 16(7): pp. 1087–1092.

[3] Shoemaker T., et al., *Reemerging Sudan Ebola virus disease in Uganda,* 2011. Emerging infectious diseases, 2012. 18(9): pp. 1480–1483.

[4] MOH, *Epidemiological report of the Ebola outbreak in Kibaale district, Report by the Ministry of Health, Uganda,* in *Sitrep Ebola,* J. Wamala, Luswa Editor 2012, Ministry of Health, Uganda: Kampala.

[5] Okware S.I., et al., *An outbreak of Ebola in Uganda.* Tropical medicine & international health: TM & IH, 2002. 7(12): pp. 1068–1075.

[6] WHO, *Ebola haemorrhagic fever in Sudan, 1976. Report of a WHO/International Study Team.* Bulletin of the World Health Organization, 1978. 56(2): pp. 247–270.

[7] WHO, *Ebola Situation Report - 28 October 2015, in ReliefWeb*2015, WHO, Geneva.

[8] McCormick J.B., et al., *Biologic differences between strains of Ebola virus from Zaire and Sudan*. The Journal of infectious diseases, 1983. 147(2): pp. 264–267.

[9] Geisbert T.W., et al., *Pathogenesis of Ebola hemorrhagic fever in cynomolgus macaques: evidence that dendritic cells are early and sustained targets of infection*. The American journal of pathology, 2003. 163(6): pp. 2347–2370.

[10] Fieldman H., *Ebola haemorrhagic fever*. Lancet, 2011. 377: pp. 849–862.

[11] Leroy E.M., et al., *Human Ebola outbreak resulting from direct exposure to fruit bats in Luebo, Democratic Republic of Congo,* 2007. Vector borne and zoonotic diseases, 2009. 9(6): pp. 723–728.

[12] Pourrut X., et al., *Large serological survey showing cocirculation of Ebola and Marburg viruses in Gabonese bat populations, and a high seroprevalence of both viruses in Rousettus aegyptiacus*. BMC infectious diseases, 2009. 9: p. 159.

[13] Ksiazek T.G., et al., *Clinical virology of Ebola hemorrhagic fever (EHF): virus, virus antigen, and IgG and IgM antibody findings among EHF patients in Kikwit, Democratic Republic of the Congo, 1995*. The Journal of infectious diseases, 1999. 179 Suppl 1: pp. S177–187.

[14] Dowell S.F., et al., *Transmission of Ebola hemorrhagic fever: a study of risk factors in family members, Kikwit, Democratic Republic of the Congo, 1995. Commission de Lutte contre les Epidemies a Kikwit*. The Journal of infectious diseases, 1999. 179 Suppl 1: pp. S87–91.

[15] Baron R.C., McCormick J.B., and Zubeir O.A., *Ebola virus disease in southern Sudan: hospital dissemination and intrafamilial spread*. Bulletin of the World Health Organization, 1983. 61(6): pp. 997–1003.

[16] UNICEF, *Humantarian action report 2007, 2007*, UNICEF Uganda: Uganda.

[17] Towner J.S., et al., *Newly discovered Ebola virus associated with hemorrhagic fever outbreak in Uganda*. PLoS pathogens, 2008. 4(11): p. e1000212.

[18] Wamala J., *Update report Ebola in Luwero Aug 2011, unpublished,* J. Wamala, Editor 2011, Ministry, Health, Uganda: Kampla.

[19] Lamunu M., et al., *Containing a haemorrhagic fever epidemic: the Ebola experience in Uganda (October 2000-January 2001)*. International journal of infectious diseases: IJID: official publication of the International Society for Infectious Diseases, 2004. 8(1): pp. 27–37.

[20] Borchert M., *Ebola haemorrhagic fever outbreak in Masindi District, Uganda: outbreak description and lessons learned*. BMC Infect Dis, 2011 11: p. 357.

[21] Bartsch S.M., Gorham K., and Lee B.Y., *The cost of an Ebola case. Pathog Glob Health*, 2015. 109(1): pp. 4–9.

[22] Szabo L., *Costs of responding toEebola adding up, in USA TODAY 2014*, USA Today: USA.

http://dx.doi.org/10.5772/63056

[23] Clark D.V., et al., *Long-term sequelae after Ebola virus disease in Bundibugyo, Uganda: a retrospective cohort study*. Lancet Infect Dis, 2015. 15(8): pp. 905–912.

[24] Wendo C., *Caring for the survivors of Uganda's Ebola epidemic one year on*. Lancet, 2001. 358(9290): p. 1350.

Chapter 2

Ebola and Health Partnerships, Action in a Time of Crisis

Colin S Brown, Mohamed Elsherbiny,
Oliver Johnson, Amardeep Kamboz, Marta Lado,
Andrew Leather, Natalie Mounter,
Suzanne Thomas, Dan Youkee, Naomi Walker,
Waheed Awonuga, TB Kamara, Cecilia Kamara,
Quaanan Kessete and Ramatu Ngauja

Additional information is available at the end of the chapter

http://dx.doi.org/10.5772/63440

Abstract

The chapter explores the role of health partnerships in delivering services throughout the West African Ebola Virus Disease epidemic, including the creation of the Ministry of Health and Sanitation, Sierra Leone, Ebola Holding Unit models, command and control structures, research into diagnostics and care pathways, and general medical care. It will highlight how this provided resilience during the Ebola response, and how this will aid health systems strengthening going forward.

Keywords: ebola, health partnership, impact, resilience, sustainable

1. Introduction to partnership working & existing health structure in Sierra Leone

In 2014, Connaught Hospital and the King's Sierra Leone Partnership (KSLP) were at the epicentre of the Ebola Virus Disease (EVD) outbreak in West Africa and, given the unprecedented nature of disease spread, had to develop new approaches to managing the clinical response. This chapter explores our model of Ebola Holding Units (EHUs) within government hospitals, including the role of international partnerships, how to maintain general health services during an outbreak and the importance of effective command and control. We discuss how to conduct research and build longer-term capacity during a crisis. We hope the chapter will be of interest to those organisations working in EVD-prone countries, as well as those interested in broader aspects of EVD resilience and outbreak response.

1.1. Connaught Hospital

Connaught Hospital is the main adult tertiary referral and teaching hospital in Sierra Leone. Established during the colonial period and located in the downtown area of the capital city, Freetown, it has 300 medical and surgical beds and a range of specialist clinics such as for human immunodeficiency virus (HIV), tuberculosis (TB) and ophthalmology. Prior to the outbreak, the hospital was operating with limited resources for many years. As a result, patients paid fees for individual services and the infrastructure, such as sinks and taps, was degraded, with limited equipment or supplies such as gloves or cannulas. The hospital had only 10 consultants, fully specialised doctors, a small number for a facility of this size, and few ward sisters. Therefore, more junior staff would have significant clinical responsibility and only limited access to supervision.

1.2. Sierra Leone context

Connaught is part of a wider government health system with about 30 hospitals and more than 1000 primary care units across a country of six million people. Despite significant progress over the last 10 years, the health system still faced major challenges before the Ebola outbreak. A colonial legacy of few health training institutions, with the county's only medical school established in 1988, was compounded by the effects of protracted civil war (1994–2002), which saw many health workers leave the country or left unable to complete their specialist training. This all contributed to a major human resource crisis, with about 150 doctors, equal to 2 doctors per 100,000 people (compared to 280 in the UK) [1], and well below World Health Organization (WHO) minimum standards [2].

The civil war also led to significant damage to health facilities across the country and undermined the capacity of key institutions that were responsible for the governance and management of health services, such as the Ministry of Health & Sanitation (MOHS). A small, albeit growing, economy resulted in low salaries for staff and limited resources to provide free drugs or services to patients. The country was heavily dependent on international donors to fund health services, both through the government and through non-governmental providers. Despite these challenges, the government had made a major commitment to health, symbolised by the launch of the Free Health Care initiative for under-5 year-old children and pregnant or lactating women in 2008.

Outside of the health systems, widespread extreme poverty resulted in poor housing, limited access to water and sanitation, low levels of formal employment and literacy, and a limited ability to pay for out-of-pocket fees for health services. There was also a strong culture of traditional beliefs and use of informal and unregulated health providers. These all had significant impacts on the burden of disease and the attitudes and behaviours of patients.

http://dx.doi.org/10.5772/63440

Overall, the consequence was poor health outcomes: a life expectancy of 46 and one of highest infant mortality rates in the world (161/1000 live births) [1].

1.3. Partnership working

In this context, Connaught Hospital invited the support of King's Health Partners (KHP) in 2012 to help strengthen the capacity of the hospital over the long term. KHP is an Academic Health Sciences Centre consisting of King's College London (KCL), in the world's top 20 university rankings, and three of the largest acute and mental health hospitals in South London. King's had over 10 years of experience of health system strengthening work in Somaliland and a strong commitment to global health.

The King's Sierra Leone Partnership was established when a small team from King's arrived at Connaught Hospital in early 2013 with the mission to help to strengthen the government health system through supporting the improvement of clinical services, training, policy and research. KSLP also partnered with the College of Medicine & Allied Health Sciences (COMAHS) and MOHS.

The King's approach was to support the hospital to implement its own improvement programme, rather than coming with an agenda. Early priorities included restructuring the Accident & Emergency Department, supporting an application for accreditation to provide postgraduate training in surgery, establishing a dental therapy training programme, reviewing management structures within the hospital and developing a regular teaching programme for junior doctors.

KSLP recruited a small international team on the ground including doctors, nurses, pharmacists, hospital managers and others, embedded within the hospital doing a mixture of clinical and technical advisory work and teaching. This team was supported by senior specialists from the UK, who supported from a distance or visited on short trips.

The partnership was founded on the principles of mutual respect and shared learning and based on supporting the hospital's own leadership and strategy. It recognised that King's had as much or more to learn and benefit from the partnership as Sierra Leonean institutions did. Its strategy was to plan over the long term, over decades rather than months or years, and focused on the structural causes of health system challenges, such as addressing the lack of postgraduate training opportunities, rather than short term fixes, for example deploying large numbers of foreign volunteers to prop-up clinical activities. In addition, the approach was holistic, recognising that a hospital is a complex system and that to improve a particular aspect of patient care you need to address a number of interlinked components at once, which might range from developing clinical protocols to training staff, refurbishing the physical environment, improving access to medical equipment and supplies, and overhauling the medical records and finance systems.

It was in this context, Connaught Hospital and KSLP found themselves on the frontline of the outbreak when the first EVD cases were identified in Freetown in July 2014, and had to radically restructure their work in order to mount an effective response to the epidemic whilst maintaining essential health services.

2. West African EVD outbreak

The 2014–2015 West African outbreak of Ebola Virus Disease was unprecedented in terms of longevity and magnitude. More than 11,300 people have died, with some 28,600 infected across seven countries [3]. Although the reservoir of EVD is unknown, it is thought to be a fruit bat [4,5]. One introduction from the animal reservoir to the West African population is likely responsible for all of the cases seen in the region [6]. It was apparent early in the outbreak that inadequate human resourcing and physical infrastructure delayed intervention in the face of exponential spread, with "each new suspected case bring[ing] an exponential increase in resources required for testing, isolation and contact tracing" [7].

2.1. Existing models of EVD control

There have been many models of EVD care facility established to redress this challenge, some traditionally used in combatting EVD outbreaks and others developed in response to the scale of the outbreak and adapted to local design. In Sierra Leone, there were three models of care that were utilised. Ebola Treatment Centres (ETCs) most closely represent the standard model of care. These were standalone units, often purpose-built by international agencies outwith government procurement processes and placed away from population hubs. They are often subdivided into suspect and confirmed wards for all patients presenting with illness suggestive of EVD. The UK government response in Sierra Leone included the construction of many of these ETCs, operated by a variety of Non-Governmental Organisations (NGOs) [8]. Community Care Centres (CCCs) were developed in response to uncontrolled spread of EVD, often in areas with limited access to other care facilities, and provided basic health care while suspect patients awaited their EVD test results, or for provision of early treatment of confirmed cases awaiting beds to become available at ETCs. Often built in repurposed structures or as collections of small tents, they were "small, low technology, mainly staffed by nurses and community health workers and can accommodate 8 to 10 (maximum 15) patients" [9]. Ebola Holding Units were constructed in existing healthcare facilities, either repurposing existing buildings or constructing standalone units within hospital grounds. They utilise local health care workers (HCWs), allowing for ongoing healthcare services to be safely delivered alongside safe isolation, testing, initial treatment and onward referral of EVD-positive patients to ETCs or ward-based or outpatient care of EVD-negative patients. They were adopted by MOHS in partnership with organisations such as KSLP, who helped establish EHUs attached to MOHS hospitals, initially at Connaught Hospital then four others. KSLP also helped other facilities prepare for EVD cases, trained local and international staff for a variety of organisations, and supported command and control structures across the Western Area of the country (the peninsula area surrounding Freetown) to harmonise referrals and transfers between units [10].

2.2. Partnership working in EVD care

In March 2014, KSLP was invited by MOHS to contribute to the national Ebola Case Management Taskforce. Utilising infectious disease experience within the in-country team, we helped

http://dx.doi.org/10.5772/63440

develop national guidelines for suspect case definition and developed safe isolation protocols for isolating and testing suspect cases across MOHS settings. KSLP staff later contributed to the WHO EVD management guidelines. The MOHS, with the support of KSLP and other international partners, started establishing EHUs at MOHS hospitals in Freetown in May 2014, before the first case of EVD in country. Initially a two-bed EHU at Connaught Hospital was opened, and as the outbreak escalated in Freetown in August 2014, KSLP and MOHS increased Connaught Hospital capacity and established four further units. We also assisted in setting up of two additional units.

The EHU model aimed to "(1) reduce cases in the local community through rapid isolation of symptomatic and suspect EVD cases to prevent onward transmission, (2) prevent nosocomial transmission through patient separation and regular decontamination of surfaces and floors, (3) improve survival of isolated patients through provision of safe EVD and non-EVD medical care, (4) maintain general healthcare through prompt diagnosis of EVD and onward transfer of patients to dedicated ETCs, alongside exclusion of EVD and triage of negative patients into outpatient or inpatient facilities for general care, allowing hospitals to remain safe and functional, even during peak EVD transmission, and (5) reducing healthcare worker infections through staff training inside the EHU and infection prevention and control strengthening on general wards, avoiding closure of facilities" [11].

Between 29th May 2014 and 19th January 2015, the five KSLP-supported MOHS EHUs (with 79 beds) had isolated a substantial proportion of the confirmed cases seen within the Western Area Urban and Rural districts (1159 of the 3097 cases). These facilities were 'front-loaded' in terms of construction of facilities, largely clustered early in the response efforts. They were cheap and quick to develop, with construction costs arriving at under $50,000 in total with one-week start-up times. We believe this model of care, detailed in Section 3 for Connaught Hospital, has significance for future outbreak control due to the rapidity of development and resilience for hospital functioning [11].

2.3. Outputs of partnership working

Within the EHU, Connaught Hospital and KSLP staff were able to validate a newly developed Rapid Diagnostic Test to prove its utility; assess the efficacy of the WHO suspect case definition, and determine whether a screening algorithm could be used prospectively to identify which suspect cases had a high likelihood of being EVD-positive; identify risk factors for mortality; assess how many patients discharged with a negative EVD-diagnosis were readmitted to any other facility in the Western Area, identifying the risk of potential infection within the EHU; and examine whether our environmental decontamination practices were effective (all Section 4). An ongoing programme of education focuses on delivering resilience within the hospitals for Intensive Care, Accident & Emergency and General Medicine and Surgery (Section 5), and Infection Prevention and Control (IPC) and Water and Sanitation (WASH) projects (Section 6) that will increase infrastructural resilience (Section 6). The command and control structures were developed alongside these operational research questions, which allowed for early harmonisation across the Freetown response and served as a model for national scale up to the district responses outside the Western Area (Section 7). We have also remodelled temporary EHUs into permanent infection diseases units, retaining capacity to isolate, test, and treat EVD along with other infectious outbreaks, now and in the future, and laboratory strengthening with assistance from Public Health England (PHE) will aim to provide the necessary capacity to diagnose and detect future outbreaks of cholera and other diseases that could mimic EVD. A dedicated Infectious Disease Centre for Excellence will bring together leaders for the purposes of training, education, research and capacity building. A cohort of local healthcare staff of all cadres has developed significant skills and experience that can be harnessed. These areas are expanded in the following sections.

3. Operations of an Ebola Holding Unit, Connaught Hospital

To better understand how partnership working enabled rapid instigation and scale-up of the Connaught Hospital response, the following section highlights the various aspects regarding developing the EHU facility.

3.1.1. Staffing

The first isolated patients were cared for by one of Connaught's three consultant medical physicians, junior medical staff and the senior nurse in charge of accident & Emergency. Following the consultant's sad death from EVD in June 2014, a small team of two or three international staff who had been working with KSLP before the EVD outbreak, took over care within the isolation facility. Over time the confidence of national hospital staff and volunteers grew and the team expanded to keep pace with the increase in bed numbers (see **Table 1**). As the number of Ebola cases in Freetown escalated the EHU expanded from an initial two bedded unit in late May 2014 bed capacity to nine, then a 16-bed unit with two additional child cots in August 2014. Consequently the operational aspects of running the unit also had to be scaled up.

Staff	Roles	Number
Caregiving staff	Admit patients and give personal/nursing care Administer medications Ensure blood sample collection by laboratory staff and check results Arrange patient transfer to ETU or discharge from EHU to hospital or home Wash bodies, collect oral swabs for testing and prepare for collection by burial team	13 (national) and 8 (international)
Cleaners	Clean EHU and patients items to prevent cross infection between patients Ensure safe disposal of waste Prepare chlorine water Wash bodies and prepare for collection by burial team	12 (national)
Security staff	Ensure public safety during patient admission or removal of corpses Liaise with visitors and relatives Ensure security of patients, staff and supplies	4 (national)

http://dx.doi.org/10.5772/63440

Staff	Roles	Number
Laboratory technicians	Collect and package blood samples Arrange transport of samples to laboratory	7 (national)
District surveillance officers	Interview patient for contact tracing Undertake contact tracing Liaise with the Command Centre to arrange transfers to ETU Liaise with relatives to discharge patients Liaise with burial team and families about dead patients	2 (national)
Screeners	Screen and identify suspected cases at the main entrance of the hospital Liaise with caregiving staff about patients requiring admission	6 (national)

Table 1. Numbers of clinical staff required for the twenty bed Ebola Holding Unit at Connaught Hospital at the height of the EVD outbreak, November 2014.

The caregiving staff, cleaners, screeners and security staff provided 24-h cover for the unit across three shifts. In order to repair and maintain the unit, some hospital maintenance staff (e.g. carpenters, electricians and plumbers) were trained in using Personal Protective Equipment (PPE) and would occasionally work in the unit under the guidance of an experienced member of staff. In addition, there was an operational team to provide support for the EHU (see **Table 2**) who were able to draw on technical advisors and an operations manager based in London for advice and assistance as required.

Staff	Roles	Number
Programme director	Overall management of EHU Liaison with partners and external agencies	1 (international)
Clinical lead—infectious diseases specialist doctor	Technical advice and clinical supervision Staff training and management Liaison with central coordinating agencies	1 (international)
Operations lead	Co-ordinate supplies, logistics and finances Staff training and management	1 (international)
Operations assistant	Assist with logistics	1 (national)
Supplies coordinator	Order and manage all supplies Staff training and management	1 (international)
Supplies assistant	Assist with supplies	2 (national)
Human resource coordinator	Recruitment of international staff In-country support for international staff	1 (international)
Senior nurse	Recruitment of national staff Management of national staff in EHU	1 (national)

Table 2. Numbers of operational staff required to support the Ebola Holding Unit at Connaught Hospital, November 2014.

3.1.2. *Equipment and supplies*

With the agreement of Connaught Hospital management, a space was identified within the hospital for use as an EHU. This was prepared jointly by international volunteers and a range of hospital staff including nurses, doctors and maintenance staff. All initial equipment was purchased locally. As the outbreak continued some specific pieces of equipment which would improve safety within the EHU but were not available locally were shipped in e.g. non touch clinical waste bins. Several features made the identified space useful to create the EHU—it was adjacent to the triage area at the front of the hospital, so any patients identified at being at risk of EVD were easily transported into the unit. There were no steps, separate entrance and exits (though the latter had to be constructed) with the capacity for unidirectional flow, and was a physical building that withstood the rigors of repeated cleaning, allowed for security, and ventilation for patients. It also was self-contained from the rest of the hospital, had its own water supply, and space for dressing areas and decontamination. Construction was relatively simple and involved building temporary doors, plastic sheets between bedspaces, wooden furniture and supplies such as buckets, cabinets to store medication, and clocks.

Availability of PPE, cleaning supplies and drugs was limited at the beginning of the outbreak and a rapid donation of essential items was sent by air freight from KHP in August 2014. As more supplies became available in Central Medical Stores (CMS), the government agency responsible for distributing healthcare supplies to hospital facilities, the majority of supplies for the EHU were requested through the government supply chain. Hospital management authorised the orders which were prepared by the supplies coordinator. This approach was adopted to reduce dependence on a parallel supply chain which could distort overall data about supply requirements. Specific items continued to be shipped in either because they were considered essential but in short supply (e.g. shoe covers and long gloves) or because they were required on safety grounds (i.e. disposable masks with visor attached). Non-medical supplies for patients (e.g. soap, bedsheets, clothes and drinking water) were sourced locally and provided through another NGO who received donor funding specifically to fulfil for this function for a number of EHUs. Storage space for all the supplies was provided by the hospital management.

3.1.3. *Safety*

To ensure safe operation of the EHU, many aspects of care were carefully negotiated with the MOHS and hospital management. Concerns regarding overflow were managed by strictly limiting bed numbers to a capacity that was deemed safe. We never accepted more patients into the EHU than we had beds available for, however we constructed a tented area outside the hospital entrance to deal with overflow where families could bring relatives awaiting admission and were provided with IPC to care for them. Early in the Western Area outbreak, when there were no EHU beds available the Accident & Emergency department was temporarily closed until spare beds became available to protect the general hospital wards. The whole hospital staff played a tremendous role in safely managing the wards during the outbreak, and morale was boosted for all healthcare staff who were given limited additional hazard payment for their work. Plastic sheeting was challenging—it was initially employed in the unit

http://dx.doi.org/10.5772/63440

to provide separation between patients, however this was taken down as IPC management was easier without having to decontaminate the plastic surfaces. Security was occasionally a concern in healthcare facilities and the Royal Sierra Leone Armed Forces were stationed at the main entrance to aid with calming measures, given the high numbers of patients presenting given Connaught was one the few functioning facilities in the Western Area. Towards the end of the outbreak, from March 2015 we started testing all inpatients for HIV. All patients who tested negative for EVD and diagnosed with HIV were linked into onward services for HIV care, and all EVD-negative patients were showered and given a clean pair of clothes before leaving the unit for onward management on the medical wards. This care was enabled by a credit provided by KSLP to pay for basic medications and tests.

3.2. Model of supervision

Building on the existing model of partnership working, the ultimate aim was to build the capacity of EHU staff to run the unit independently in the future.

At the beginning of the outbreak fear of infection, lack of training and lack of resources were the main reasons for hospital staff being unwilling to work in EHUs. In order to address these issues international staff provided practical training and ongoing supervision. The role and importance of standard operating procedures was emphasised regularly to minimise HCW infection. Role modelling was an important factor in building the confidence of new staff. This helped consolidate the adoption of the correct procedures by new staff and built confidence in the safety of those procedures. For that reason international staff were recruited on the understanding that they would be expected to perform the same duties as all other staff. Development of a responsive supply chain for the unit also helped to maintain staff commitment. As the numbers and competency of the national staff increased, the numbers of international staff decreased significantly so that by the end of the outbreak only one international clinician was on-call to assist with clinical issues. The management of supplies from CMS was handed over to the hospital pharmacy and storekeeper.

Good working relationships with the Matron and the Senior Nurse in the Emergency Department were critical for the recruitment, management and disciplining of EHU staff. An identified team leader for each shift strengthened communication between staff.

One challenge was the stigma experienced by those working inside the EHU from relatives and colleagues. There were reports of workers being shunned by other health workers or expelled from their houses by their families. It was important to acknowledge these difficulties with staff in the early stages of training and discuss contingency plans for dealing with these challenges.

All staff working inside the EHU were entitled to a risk allowance which was distributed by the National Ebola Response Centre (NERC). There were often problems in the access to this financial incentive, and KSLP provided a smaller performance related bonus (based on a written report of attendance, performance and safety while working) in addition to this allowance which was an effective tool for providing feedback and incentive for good performance. However at other EHUs, this was not attempted, and good mentorship and encouragement were sufficient to motivate local staff.

3.3. Using the Connaught Hospital EHU as a training hub

Training was one of the KSLP pillars of work during the outbreak. After setting up the Connaught EHU, the first in the Western Area for suspected EVD cases, KSLP developed a training method used to train more than 400 health care workers, international and national, to work in EHUs and ETCs.

3.3.1. Model of training

The training groups were structured in small groups of trainees (between 6 and 10 people per group subdivided into small teams of between 3 and 5 members). It was important to ensure that the training was practical, interactive and with opportunities for the students to engage with the live environment and implement what they had learnt in lectures with direct supervision from the trainer.

All staff working in patient areas received the three-phase training described below (see **Figure 1**). Before starting clinical work, all staff had to complete Phase 1 and Phase 2 training. See **Table 3** for an example of training timetable for Phases 1 and 2.

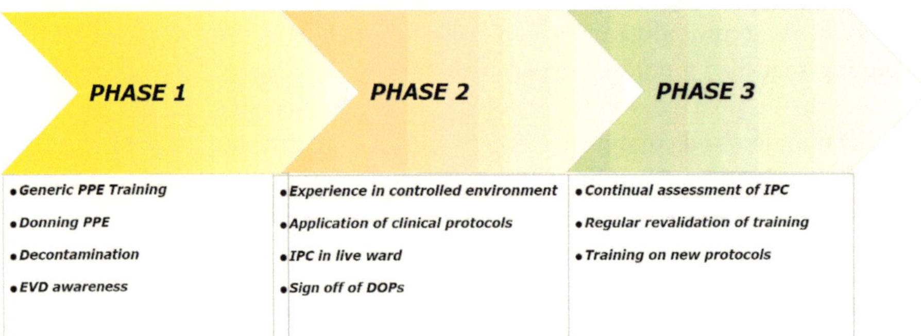

Figure 1. Three phase training model at Connaught Hospital Ebola Holding Unit.

Day 1—Phase 1		
AM	General induction and orientation	Conference room
PM	Training session 1	Conference room followed by isolation unit
	• Ebola	
	• Connaught isolation unit	
	• Infection prevention	

http://dx.doi.org/10.5772/63440

Day 1—Phase 1		
	✤ Hand hygiene	
	✤ PPE dressing and undressing	
	✤ Cleaning and waste management	
	• Tour of the isolation unit	
Day 2—Phase 1 followed by start of Phase 2		
AM	Training session 2: isolation unit standard operating procedures	Conference room
PM	Training session 3: practical training	Isolation unit
	• Standard operating procedures	
	• Chlorine preparation	
	Case discussions	
Day 3—Phase 2		
AM/PM	Practical training	Isolation unit

Table 3. Example Timetable for Phases 1 and 2.

Phase 1 consisted of generic EVD training, including basic PPE training, decontamination procedures, IPC protocols and basic knowledge and awareness of EVD. The method was based on theoretical lectures and included the principles of the construction and setting up of an isolation unit according to the WHO and Médecins Sans Frontières guidelines.

Phase 2 focused on the application of protocols to the real life environment. Training took place within the Connaught EHU, and was provided by experienced staff who ensured adequate supervision. Throughout Phase 2, there was a gradual increase in both time spent inside the unit and procedures performed by trainees. Direct observation of procedural skills (DOPs) was used to assess competence. These practical lessons were developed inside the EHU with real patients and different scenarios to help the trainees to understand and put in practice the best clinical management with EVD patients.

Phase 3 training was provided within their own EHU. Staff were formally revalidated in their decontamination procedures and IPC protocols on a regular basis. See **Figure 2** for an example of an assessment tool used for revalidation. All staff were retrained as new procedures or protocols were adopted. In many training sessions, direct explanations and advice in storage, supplies of consumables and PPE were also provided, based on the experiences gained at Connaught Hospital, with the aim of assisting in the setting up of new units at government facilities in the Western Area and all over the country through other partners [12].

Phase 4, the newest training phase, was established after Sierra Leone was declared EVD-free. It allows EVD-healthcare workers to receive updates and refreshment of previously deployed EVD training to ensure readiness when new cases arise. Currently, KSLP is developing updated training for HCWs that is focused on lessons learnt from the outbreak, mainly based

Removing PPE

Step	Achieved	Comments
1. Stand in chlorine footbath at the entrance of the room for one minute.		
2. Wash gloved hands with water and soap (**First bucket**).		
3. Wash gloved hands in 0.5% chlorine solution for one minute (**Second bucket**).		
4. Remove apron by grasping at sides and holding away from you deposit in bin.		
5. Wash gloved hands in 0.5% chlorine solution for one minute (**Second bucket**).		
6. Remove outer gloves and deposit in bin		
7. Wash gloved hands in 0.5% chlorine solution for thirty seconds (**Third bucket**).		
8. Looking in mirror take zip of PPE suit between thumb and forefinger of one hand and undo. Grasp hood of suit and pull off head. Roll suit down, touching as little as possible.		
9. Wash gloved hands in 0.5% chlorine solution for thirty seconds (**Third bucket**).		
10. Looking in mirror remove face shield.		
11. Wash gloved hands in 0.5% chlorine solution for thirty seconds (**Third bucket**).		
12. Remove inner gloves.		
13. Wash hands in 0.05% chlorine solution for one minute (**Fourth bucket**).		
14. Proceed to chlorine footbath for one minute.		
15. Put on gloves.		
16. Remove boots and place in boot rack, put on shoes.		
17. Remove gloves.		
18. Wash hands with water and soap (**Fifth bucket**).		
19. Leave isolation unit through back door.		
20. Wash hands with soap and water outside the clinical office.		

Figure 2. Staff PPE competency assessment tool used during phase 3 training.

http://dx.doi.org/10.5772/63440

in case management and care of the patients with actors and different scenarios inside the EHU, e.g. management of sepsis, and of confused and agitated patients. It also includes an update in IPC and special situations such as pregnant EVD patients. This training is also oriented to prepare trainers to deliver this material to more HCWs to ensure onward resilience. **Table 4** details an example timetable for this phase.

Day 1		
AM	Refresher training in	Conference room
	• Ebola	
	• EVD clinical management	
	• IPC updates	
	• Training skills (for those who will be trainers)	
PM	• Clinical cases	Conference room
	• Simulation scenarios in the isolation unit	Isolation unit
		Conference room
	• Pregnancy in EVD patients	

Table 4. Example timetable for Phase 4.

4. Prioritising research in the EVD outbreak setting: the role of health partnerships

The scale and duration of the West African EVD outbreak provided a unique opportunity to study the clinical features and management of EVD to generate evidence for best practice. Prior to this outbreak, case management was based on expert opinion and evidence from limited case studies and small patient cohorts in Central and East Africa [13–16]. Several KSLP clinical volunteers and senior Connaught medical staff had research expertise. However, significant barriers to undertaking research existed. There was a shortage of staff to deliver basic clinical care for much of the outbreak. Upholding high standards of ethical conduct and governance was essential, but many of the clinicians (doctors and nurses) working in the EHU had not received prior training in research methodology and the necessary training and associated research governance processes required considerable time and effort to set up.

4.1.1. The importance of research in an outbreak setting

In this context, we focused our efforts on standardising best clinical practice and carefully recording important clinical information so that retrospective analysis could be performed. We prioritised questions that would influence patient management and interrogated our clinical dataset for the answers. In doing this, we felt we could generate evidence to improve wider practice, whilst continuing our focus on care at an individual level.

4.1.2. What were the important research questions?

Identification of suspected clinical cases for isolation and EVD testing was a critical step in EVD outbreak control. We noticed that despite applying the consensus case definition to all admissions at Connaught Hospital, several inpatients who became unwell and were later found to have EVD, did not meet the suspected case definition at presentation, and therefore potentially exposed nursing staff and other patients on general wards. Other individuals may have remained in the community, putting friends and family at risk of EVD. Effective screening of suspected cases was identified as a critical part of the patient pathway that was liable to impede EVD outbreak control.

Additionally, we struggled with lack of capacity in our facility. Despite increasing the number of Connaught EHU beds, we frequently had patients waiting outside the hospital for space to become available due to high transmission in the community. Our capacity was limited by duration of stay, proportional to the time required to obtain an EVD test result. Once a patient was admitted, a blood sample was collected for EVD testing and transported to centralised specialist laboratory for EVD polymerase chain reaction (PCR) testing. The PCR assay required technical skill and advanced laboratory equipment and turnaround time ranged from 1 to 7 days. We could not discharge or transfer patients until their results were available. It became apparent that a point-of-care test with a high sensitivity and a reasonable specificity would transform our case management, allowing us to discharge negative patients with confidence, freeing up beds for new suspected cases, and increasing our admission rate.

4.1.3. Operational research around data management and EHU safety

Clinical information was collected daily from patients admitted to the EHU using a standardised proforma, by clinicians and district surveillance officers. This included demographic data of patients including contact details and travel history, symptoms on admission, date of admission and symptom onset, source of admission, specimen collection date and time, laboratory result and patient outcome i.e. whether the patient was discharged home, transferred to the wards, referred to an ETC or died. This information was then entered into a database in Microsoft Excel, which was used to analyse the data.

In several instances, the information gathered was used to improve the quality of care and to identify bottlenecks in the management of patients in the isolation unit. For instance, a retrospective cohort study of presenting features of EVD confirmed our suspicion that case definitions were not sensitive enough, that baseline symptoms were poor at discriminating EVD-positive cases from other illnesses, and supported the implementation of rapid diagnostic testing [17]. These findings were published open-access in July 2015. The number of hours/days taken to send the blood sample to the laboratory and the time taken to get the results back was analysed to identify delays for targeted interventions, including reorganisation of the laboratory transport system. Delays in turnaround led to increased length of stay and delays in public health action such as contact tracing, highlighting that up-to-date real-time operational data is critical to optimise resource allocation and response [18]. When concerns about nosocomial transmission within the isolation unit were raised, we were able to demonstrate that this was infrequent, by examining the frequency of readmissions (amongst patients

http://dx.doi.org/10.5772/63440

who tested negative and were discharged), which was low. We identified a maximum positive readmission rate of 3.3% [19], lower than has been previously reported [20].

These findings support the EHU model as a safe method for isolation of suspect EVD patients and their role in limiting the spread of EVD, and will be very important in the coordination and implementation of a response to any future outbreak of EVD. Further operational research was conducted within the EHU to inform decontamination practices, as evidence was lacking. We conducted an audit of decontamination procedures inside Connaught Hospital EHU, showing that prior to decontamination, Ebola virus RNA was detected by PCR within a limited area at all bedside sites tested, but not at sites distant to the bedside. Following decontamination, few areas contained detectable Ebola virus RNA, however in areas beneath bedspaces there was evidence of transfer of Ebola virus material during cleaning. By retraining of cleaning staff (outlined in Section 3) we saw reduced evidence of environmental contamination after decontamination, highlighting that regular refresher training is essential during the course of EVD outbreaks [21].

4.2. Case study—evaluating a point-of-care rapid diagnostic test for EVD

We conducted a study assessing the diagnostic accuracy of a new point-of-care test (RDT) against the gold-standard EVD PCR assay. The RDT test had been developed by the UK Defence Science Technology Laboratories and was delivered to us by PHE who had constructed laboratories in the Western Area. We received 300 prototypes for evaluation. The new test required only one drop of capillary blood generated from a single finger-prick (compared to several millilitres of peripheral venous blood for the standard test). The result was generated by a lateral flow device at the site of testing within 20 min. We designed a diagnostic accuracy study to evaluate the test in an operational setting. Clinical staff who provided care for patients in KSLP-supported units were trained in the study procedure and use of the new test, and tested all admissions to their isolation units with suspected EVD, following informed consent. Phlebotomists who would routinely collect venous blood from all admissions for standard EVD testing by PCR continued to do so. Therefore, all patients enrolled in the study received two tests (the new unproven RDT test) and the routine (gold standard) test. At the end of the study, we were able to compare the performance of the new test with the routine test and estimate the sensitivity, specificity, positive and negative predictive values. The study was implemented in early 2015, in four KSLP-supported clinical sites. The incidence of EVD in Freetown was rapidly decreasing during this time but despite this, the study recruited 138 participants. The test proved highly sensitive and specific and was published in an open access peer-reviewed journal, within two months of study completion [22].

4.2.1. Research governance

There were ethical and governance issues to consider with the sensitive nature of the information that was being collected. Patients were assured of confidentiality and anonymity and permission for the research database was sought from of the Medical Superintendent of Connaught Hospital. The purpose, objectives and method of data collection were explained to all four Medical superintendents, who allowed the study to take place. The study had institutional approval at all sites and received prospective approval of the Sierra Leone Ethics and Scientific Review Committee.

4.2.2. Challenges in study implementation

A major challenge to study implementation was human resources. Few staff were willing to have direct patient contact, and these staff were overwhelmed by the demands of delivering essential clinical care under challenging circumstances. Working conditions inside the EHU were difficult, with full PPE required at all times and exemplary infection control as per the Phased Training (Section 3).

Patient notes were kept outside the unit, as records inside could not be removed. For data entry, these were inputted in batches after the patient had been discharged, which was time-consuming given the high turnover of patients. A major challenge was forms with incomplete data, and source documents (admission logs and laboratory records) were required to fill in gaps. The RDT result was documented inside the unit and then called out to staff outside. Patient study information leaflets were kept inside the EHU, but destroyed on discharge. A fresh copy was given to patients who were discharged to take away with them. Verbal, rather than written informed consent was taken from patients. Staff documented the process by signing a log outside the EHU.

All staff working on the RDT study offered their time voluntarily, and the study received no specific funding. There were no financial incentives for staff or patients to engage with research and whilst there was enthusiasm amongst staff to be trained in research methods and to assist with the development of an RDT, this diminished once the practicalities became apparent. Taking consent and performing the test required extra time inside the EHU and some staff felt they should be financially compensated for this. Government payments for clinical work had been delayed and some staff were suffering considerable financial hardship and low morale, as described in Section 3.

The RDT study protocol required amendment to routine sample transport and processing policies and some clinical and technical staff expressed (not unfounded) concern that this would negatively impact on patient care. These concerns were addressed by the local ethical and institutional boards and the study was conducted in adherence to international standards of research practice. However, despite this there was some reluctance to support the study and instances in which this resulted in protocol interference.

4.3. Lessons learned

Recognising staff participation in clinical research was important. Certificates of achievement were produced and were popular. An experienced full time study coordinator at each study site would have been effective at encouraging staff and patient participation, and financial incentives for staff would probably have been more effective. However as with routine clinical work, leadership by example of an experienced individual was the most effective way to improve staff morale and motivation.

Communication was extremely important at all levels. Firstly, more widespread consultation with hospital, clinic and laboratory staff about research protocols prior to decisions to implement them would have been beneficial. Decisions tended to be taken at senior level without dissemination to those in key management positions on the ground and this caused misunderstandings. Training of staff in good clinical practice and research governance was vital, and as few had prior experience close supervision and re-training was necessary. Communication with patients about research was essential. We took time to do this and felt that it was effective.

With respect to the clinical database, more detailed training of the screeners on how to fill forms completely would have been beneficial and may have improved efficiency at data entry level. Automating entries into the Excel spreadsheet would have further minimised typographical errors. Innovative technologies to improve data capture inside the unit would have helped, had they been available. Various methods were considered and some were tried e.g. the use of intercoms, photography and wireless transfer of electronic records, although none were sufficiently accessible at peak of the outbreak to make a significant impact.

One strategy to address the shortage of research staff was recruitment of medical students as volunteers, who were available as the medical school was closed. This was extremely beneficial and provided the students with experience in research methods.

Despite the demonstrated accuracy of the RDT and rapid publication, the RDT is still not widely or commercially available. Lack of financial and institutional endorsement may have delayed this, and we have learned that is not sufficient to generate evidence, we must also campaign for this work to be recognised and petition for translation into improved patient care.

As a health partnership involving KHP and Connaught staff delivering and supporting clinical care for patients with suspected EVD, we were ideally placed to address important clinical research questions. Undertaking research training addressed the partnership aim of health system strengthening. However, considerable challenges existed in terms of lack of time and human resources. We addressed this by strengthening clinical data collection, which was an essential part of routine clinical care and undertaking operational research studies that we felt would have early translational impact, as detailed above.

5. General hospital functioning

Throughout the epidemic, and in particular following the death of one of the three consultant medical physicians at Connaught Hospital, a senior British medical physician volunteering with KSLP assisted the two remaining consultant physicians through providing consultant-led ward rounds and medical student teaching. He became an integral part of the delivering clinical supervision, assisting in patient management and safety, and providing valuable ongoing training opportunities for junior medical staff [22]. This was particularly important as all school and university level education was suspended in Sierra Leone for a full year.

Internal audits of tuberculosis and HIV services showed a limited reduction in number of attendances of existing and new suspect cases, and medical inpatient numbers decreased by up to half during the early outbreak [23]. Surgical cases, sadly influenced by the death of two hospital surgical staff including the country's only trauma surgeon, dramatically dropped in August 2014, and fell to 3% of expected activity [24]. This was on a background of existing shortages in "all aspects of infrastructure, personnel, and supplies required for delivering surgical care in Sierra Leone" [25]. Despite this drop in outpatient and inpatient attendance, the hospital remained open for the duration of the outbreak, in contrast to the major referral hospitals in Guinea and Liberia, and medical wards were very busy alongside the work in the EHU. The partnership approach between COHMAS, KSLP and Connaught allowed for ongoing clinical care and training of HCWs, and all aspects of Connaught Hospital are now fully operational.

As part of reconfiguration of Accident & Emergency services KSLP assisted Connaught Hospital in establishing an effective triage system, provision of free emergency treatment and improving medical record keeping within the Emergency Department. Though Emergency department attendance was negatively correlated with the local prevalence of Ebola virus disease from June 2014-June 2015, possibly due to changes in health-seeking behaviour due to fear of EVD, it remained one of the only facilities in the country where people could access non-EVD medical care [26].

Senior infectious disease staff from KSLP were engaged in the revision of the national TB and HIV guidelines, and the TB clinic was temporarily relocated to new premises, allowing for the construction of a dedicated infectious diseases unit that can be utilised for safe isolation of patients in future highly infectious outbreaks such as cholera.

6. Water, sanitation and hygiene (WASH), infection prevention & control (IPC), and general hospital functioning

6.1.1. Background to IPC in Sierra Leone

IPC was not a known term in Sierra Leone until the recovery phase of the epidemic and there were no dedicated IPC specialists at hospital or national level. IPC was not an element of medical or nursing undergraduate training nor was there any IPC training provided by hospital facilities. Poor IPC practices within healthcare facilities have been attributed as one reason why Ebola outbreaks propagate including that seen in West Africa [27–30] and are a contributing factor in the high rate of HCW infections seen in Sierra Leone [31]. It was clear that the establishment of IPC in Sierra Leone had to be a key part of the postepidemic recovery plan that would help protect against another outbreak. Major factors affecting the proper implementation of IPC included: lack of IPC infrastructure, appropriate PPE and other essential supplies at healthcare facilities, and hand hygiene stations, and poor WASH infrastructure, inadequate systems for medical waste disposal, limited concepts of screening or triage, a lack of IPC knowledge among HCWs, and no IPC policies.

http://dx.doi.org/10.5772/63440

6.1.2. IPC post-EVD epidemic

In the wake of the epidemic, with funding and technical assistance from the US Centres for Disease Control and Prevention and as part of the Presidential Recovery Plan for Ebola, a large national IPC Project was started in Sierra Leone, covering all MOHS public health units and hospital facilities, titled 'IPC in Hospitals Program'. The 12-month project began in March 2015 and the first stages involved constructing an IPC infrastructure within the country, from national to facility level.

A National IPC Coordinator was appointed and the National IPC Unit was established, based at MOHS. Two national IPC policies were drawn up: one for use during an outbreak of Ebola and one for use once in non-epidemic times. Each hospital appointed a MOHS staff member as an IPC Focal Person who would be responsible for IPC within their facility. Each of these Focal Persons was supported by an NGO worker, known as an IPC Mentor. KSLP allocated IPC mentors to four different facilities in Freetown, including one to Connaught Hospital—these Mentors were international clinicians with a specific background in IPC. All of the IPC Focal Persons and IPC Mentors were sent on a specialist 2-week IPC training course to give them the specialist knowledge required to induct them into their new roles.

KSLP became a member of the Ebola Response Consortium (ERC), who gathered together the majority of partners involved in the project, enabling them to guide and monitor progress as well as instigate consistency among partners in the implementation of different stages of the project.

6.2. Establishing IPC at Connaught Hospital

The IPC team at Connaught was made up of an IPC Focal Person, IPC deputy and IPC NGO Mentor. KSLP also recruited an IPC Project coordinator who oversaw the project across the four hospital sites.

The newly formed Connaught IPC Team included an IPC Focal Person and appointed IPC Deputy who had extensive clinical and leadership experience within the hospital system and good working relationships with staff and management, liaison with MOHS, and specific IPC issues within their hospital. The KSLP IPC Mentor had a specific background and extensive training in infection control and technical knowledge and practical experience to help implement the project. Together this combination of skills and experience within the team was key to improving IPC within the hospital. We garnered support from the Medical Superintendent, Matron, and departmental managers. The IPC Focal Person always chaired and arranged these meetings, as it was essential she was recognised as the central manager for IPC at Connaught.

With over 800 workers at the hospital and a physically large facility, the IPC team established a system of IPC link persons in each clinical department, as recommended by the KSLP IPC Mentor. These were mostly nurses selected by their managers to be advocates for IPC on the wards and other clinical areas, attend regular IPC meetings and to monitor and report relevant problems to the IPC team. A Patient Safety Committee was established, comprising of heads of departments that were relevant to IPC practice and implementation, such as the environmental services department, supplies manager, Matron, Medical Superintendent, senior ward managers, and representatives from high risk areas such as the laboratory, theatres and the Infectious Diseases Unit. The IPC Focal person always chaired the meetings and guided the agenda as it was essential to establish her as the key person for IPC across the hospital.

There were several key areas that the team worked on to improve IPC within the hospital, detailed below with examples of how we used partnership working to improve the IPC system at the facility.

6.2.1. Supplies

The IPC project highlighted a long-standing national problem of lack of essential supplies and an inadequate national supplies system. Vital items such as examination gloves, bin bags, sharps containers, liquid hand soap and hand sanitiser had always been in short supply or not supplied before or during the outbreak.

The first stage of the IPC in Hospitals Program trained all staff in key IPC elements including hand washing, how and when to use and dispose of PPE, waste segregation and sharps disposal. The Connaught IPC team were aware that the theoretical training would be less effective if staff were not able to fully employ what they had learnt due to lack of supplies in clinical areas. The IPC Team therefore decided to withhold training until they first established the appropriate facilities and supplies to aid implementation of IPC practices.

The hospital staff had long been used to poor access to essential supplies and the KSLP IPC Mentor and IPC Focal Person determined the best way to improve the internal supply chain. The IPC Team used KSLP connections to liaise with and highlight supply problems to the CMS, and linked with other NGOs to see how they tackled supply issues. The IPC Focal Person and deputy used their own status and networks within MOHS to try to address existing problems.

It was vital to establish long-term sustainability within systems and also to ensure that safe practices were maintained, particularly during the tail of the EVD epidemic: this often presented a challenge with supplies. When essential supplies were not received through national procurement, KSLP resolved to provide supplies in the interim, but worked with hospital management to establish a plan of providing supplies in the long term. This strategy was effective and within two months the hospital was procuring essential IPC supplies independently. The improvements seen were due to the efforts of the management and IPC Focal Person, with encouragement and support from KSLP, to redress the problems surrounding long-term provision of supplies.

6.2.2. Training

Under guidance from the IPC in Hospitals Program, the Connaught IPC team set about training every HCW in relevant IPC aspects. Although HCWs in Sierra Leone had training during the outbreak, this was always focused on EVD and PPE, and not on more general aspects. Therefore, this was the first universal training of its kind in Sierra Leone and plans to involve all HCWs across the country were produced.

http://dx.doi.org/10.5772/63440

At Connaught, as with most institutions in the country, there is difficulty accessing lists of all relevant department employees, however after advertising the training the IPC Focal Person was able to organise attendees into the appropriate sessions. The team established two separate curricula for clinical and non-clinical staff. The IPC Focal Person and deputy highlighted specific IPC problems that clinical staff encountered and targeted the training around this, with the IPC Mentor giving guidance on specific technical areas. The non-clinical staff training presented a challenge as most participants were illiterate so the IPC team adapted training materials and used non-written assessment during the course. All team members were keen on pre- and postcourse testing for participants: the IPC Focal Person was clear that without assessment many would not study and attend all aspects of the course. The KSLP IPC mentor was aware of the valuable data that could be gathered from this training, and helped design appropriate tests, with the IPC Focal Person advising on what language was appropriate to use, the academic level of the participants and the types of questions that trainees would understand. The test was used to determine if participants should pass the training course and we shared resulting data with the hospital Monitoring and Evaluation department, the ERC, and relevant donors to help them understand IPC knowledge within the facility and the effectiveness of the training program.

6.3. WASH

As with many hospitals in Sierra Leone, there were occasional shortages of running water, and a lack of working sinks and taps, flushing toilets and functioning showers within Connaught, and it was clear that improved WASH infrastructure would have a direct impact on IPC practices within the hospital. It made IPC more implementable, and the sense of improvement and investment in hospital infrastructure raised HCW morale that subsequently increased enthusiasm for the project and improved IPC practice. With the involvement of the hospital management and the IPC team, we engaged an external contractor to work on WASH infrastructure and this was monitored and evaluated by KSLP, the ERC, MOHS and the President's office with regular updates given to Connaught senior management. In order to ensure longevity, new fixtures and fittings were procured internationally. The IPC team was keen to ensure that the fixtures would be properly maintained as they could not be easily replaced. KSLP management and the IPC team liaised with Connaught management and together we gave responsibility to the heads of each clinical department for the new fixtures and fittings in their area and ensured that they worked with the IPC team and regularly monitored WASH facilities. This provided a sense of responsibility and ownership from the clinical areas to ensure fittings were properly cared for. Successes outside of WASH included the construction of a building housing a new oxygen plant within Connaught Hospital.

6.4. Ward assessments

It was clear to the IPC Mentor and IPC Coordinator that there would need to be documented evidence of positive behaviour change and improved practice to submit to donors, the MOHS and the President's Office. The local IPC staff were not familiar with the concept of observational audits, assessing routine practice and data reporting but were quick to grasp the concept when it became clear how useful it would be to project implementation. The IPC Mentor designed an initial ward assessment and audit tool and the local IPC staff were able to give input into what were the specific ward problems and how they should be monitored. The ERC were keen to develop national ward monitoring, and Connaught's assessment tool was used as the basis of the national tool given its success. Local members of the IPC team harnessed a competitive nature among staff through weekly and monthly IPC competitions based on the results of the ward assessments, with initial prizes and scores displayed in public areas around Connaught. This remains one of the most effective ways of improving IPC practice in the hospital, though early prizes were discontinued as it was felt this was not sustainable or desirable.

6.5. Ongoing IPC at Connaught

The focus on sustainability, partnership and knowledge-sharing meant that before the end of the project, the team established an ongoing IPC system within the hospital involving regular training, link nurse meetings, sustainable supply chains and regular ward monitoring with a focus on constant improvement and evidence based practice. With this in place, Connaught, as the main tertiary hospital in the country, can further develop to become a model for the IPC in Hospitals program and for other institutions hoping to improve their own IPC practice and systems.

7. Command centre

In September 2014, KSLP assisted the District Health Management Team (DHMT) for the Western Area in building a Command Centre, as a result of an emerging need to integrate a growing number of KSLP (and other) EHUs within the wider Ebola response, and to create robust systems to direct the flow of cases from the community to EHUs, and from EHUs to ETCs. Before this time, there was a major perceived risk of EHUs overflowing (with concomitant risks to the safety of health care workers and patients), little was known of the number of suspect and probable cases within the Western Area, and there was no co-ordinated system for the transfer of suspect and positive EVD cases. With the support of KSLP, the Command Centre:

- Created a system of real-time case-identification and reporting of suspect cases by ensuring that alerts from the national alerts hotline were conveyed to a Disease Surveillance Officer (DSO) as soon as received (within daylight hours), and that DSOs alerted the Command Centre as soon as a suspect met the case definition
- Tracked in real time the number of beds available in EHUs to ensure that cases were distributed according to space and facilities did not incur the risk of overflow, and to ensure that every available bed was filled
- Created a system of ambulance co-ordination to enable the transfer of suspect EVD cases from the community into EHUs, from EHUs already at capacity into other EHUs, and EVD-positive patients to ETCs

http://dx.doi.org/10.5772/63440

- Created a central database of all suspect EVD cases, updated with final outcomes, and maintained a live master list of all suspect EVD cases awaiting transfer to an EHU
- Collated laboratory results and communicated these results with facilities that could not access or did not have the capacity to ascertain their own results.

7.1.1. Systems

All systems were either paper based, using simple spreadsheets or using whiteboards, and most operations were carried out by phone and SMS—systems that could be easily be understood and learnt.

In the absence of technological resources, large whiteboards were set out around the Command Centre to enable to whole team to track operations. These detailed the following:

1. Case board: Names, addresses and contact details of all identified EVD suspect cases, their unique case ID, their location, known exposure to EVD, clinical symptoms, and risk factors and the priority category they belonged to for transfer. Also logged on this board was which facility they were assigned to, the status of their collection by ambulance (updated live), and the ambulance team assigned to their collection
2. Capacity board: Bed capacity of all EHUs and ETCs, and beds available to the Command Centre for the transfer of cases by ambulance (all facilities ensure adequate space for walk-in cases). This whiteboard was updated live to reflect the changes in bed capacity throughout the day as cases were transferred.
3. Ambulance board: The number of functional vehicles, names and contact details of all ambulance staff, assigned into numbered teams, their starting location, destination and time of dispatch.
4. Map of Western Area: The location of all suspect EVD cases pinned on a map in order to determine the closest available facility and to identify potential hotspots.

7.1.2. Early operations

The early stages of set-up of the Command Centre at the DHMT, and particularly the presence of an international NGO embedded within in a government organisation, required a great deal of sensitivity to the enormous pressure the DHMT was under to respond to the rapidly growing numbers of cases in the Western Area. One of the key aims of the Command Centre was to create an objective referral system that regulated strictly prevented the overflow of the already severely limited capacity of existing EHUs and ETCs. Severe shortages of beds, ambulances, training and other resources meant that a majority of EVD-suspect cases could not be moved from their homes within 24 h. The first weeks of Command Centre operations drew attention to acute gaps in the response and the need for a rapid scale up of resources, capacity and services, such as co-ordinated ambulance, laboratory and burial services; the need for specific EVD-related services for special populations (pregnant women, neo-nates and children, those with mental health needs); better co-ordination between pillars and partners on district and national levels; better allocation and prioritisation of resources and the formation of consistent strategic policy.

Whilst data generated by the Command Centre called immediate attention to both the severity of the outbreak in the Western Area and the acute lack of resources available to mount a robust response, it was also perceived to reflect adversely on the DHMT's management of the response. KSLP remained aware of the DHMT's concerns, and tried to ensure that its relationship with the DHMT was both supporting and supportive, both operationally and in public. However, such issues highlighted how essential it was to ensure that the Command Centre was represented by a trusted figurehead with thorough knowledge of national context and good relationships with local and national government bodies, who could actively promote Command Centre operations but also resolve sensitive issues diplomatically. In the absence of such a figure during the early response period, KSLP, as the external partner helping build the Command Centre systems was continually at risk of being perceived as an undermining force.

7.1.3. Evolution

As a result of reporting from the Command Centre, in November 2014, with support from the Government of Sierra Leone and international donors, a NERC was built to ensure co-ordination and implementation of strategy and resources at national scale, to oversee Ebola Response Centres in each District (DERC). A DERC comprised of surveillance, case management, burial, quarantine, laboratory sample co-ordination and protection cells. The DERC model, which began in the Western Area and which evolved directly from operations at the DHMT Command Centre, was implemented across the country, with adaptations in line with the needs and requirements of each district.

Having assisted with the migration of the DHMT Command Centre and its functions into this new structure, KSLPs work within the DERC in the Western Area continued to focus primarily on the 'Live Case Management' cell, with a rapidly expanded team of national volunteers, who were by this time well-trained in the core processes outlined above.

7.2. Staffing

Staffing of the Live Case Management Cell were divided into five 'teams' in a flat structure under a co-ordinator who was ultimately responsible for overseeing day-to-day operations of the cell:.

Chief functions of each team were as follows:

- Case management: focal point for all EHUs and ETCs; determine bed occupancy and availability for transfers and track on whiteboards; communication of lab results, determine the movement of suspect and positive EVD cases, track and record details of patients across all units and their outcomes
- Fleet management: Manage the maintenance, fuelling and supply of ambulances, ambulance staff rotas

- Ambulance co-ordination: Dispatch and live tracking of ambulance teams, communication of ETAs to facilities
- Communications: focal point for Disease Surveillance Officers; record information of suspect cases into logs and on whiteboards; prioritise case collection according to scoring system (see Section 7.1); highlight unique risk factors or circumstances to Case Management and Ambulance Co-ordinations teams
- Data: Maintain central database of cases, aggregation and analysis of data according to reporting requirements, release daily and weekly reports as required, track KPIs

7.3. Case prioritisation

Still with an acute shortage of beds, KSLP introduced an accessible, public health-based scoring system to prioritise collection of suspect EVD cases based on their clinical state, whether they were from a home that was already quarantined, the number of people residing in the household, and their vulnerability, e.g. children under 15 who were alone, cases in public places, cases with known or perceived mental health issues.

7.4. Co-ordination

A rapid scale up of EHUs and ETCs across the Western Area began in November 2014. The Live Case Management cell, with KSLP support, became the focal point for co-ordinating and monitoring the safe opening of these facilities, ensuring each facility fully integrated with DERC systems and processes. This rapid expansion also signalled a greater need for co-ordination between EHUs and ETCs, which led to the introduction of weekly meetings, led by KSLP. These meetings became a valuable forum for updating partners on the wider picture of the response, assessing outbreak trends, for discussing daily clinical challenges, and for providing a vital feedback loop for the Live Case Management Cells on their operations. With King's support, a 'scorecard' system based on the throughput of patients through facilities, was produced and presented to all facility representatives at these meetings, which incentivised lower performing facilities to quickly resolve bottlenecks that hindered optimal throughput.

7.5. Reporting

KSLP's more targeted support to the Live Case Management Cell included developing existing capacity within the data team to generate sophisticated reports from their main database (a simple but extensive spreadsheet). As a result of KSLP's assistance in this area, by January 2015 the data team within the Cell were able to:

- Generate daily reports with Key Performance Indicators (KPIs) such as percentage occupancy of holding and treatment beds, the percentage of suspect EVD cases attended to within a 24-h period, and the inflow and outflow of cases through EHUs and into ETCs.

Such KPIs facilitated tailored decision making at strategic levels of the response, for example EHU and ETC expansion was planned according to need, and additional resources were allocated as needed to ensure that suspect EVD cases were responded to within a 24-h period.

- Develop metrics to assess case flow from the time of identification of a suspect case by a DSO, through to discharge (if EVD-negative) or to ETC (if EVD-positive). These metrics were crucial in assessing the throughput of cases through facilities, identifying bottlenecks in the system, and enabling facilities to assess and optimise their own performance (see **Figure 3**). The optimal throughput target was for a suspect EVD case to be tested and either discharged or transferred to an ETC within 24 h of admission.
- Collect and aggregate simple clinical data such as fatality rates and rates of discharge across EHU and ETCs for use by EHUs, ETCs and epidemiological partners.
- Assess and aggregate the number of EVD suspect cases admitted to EHUs via notification to the national hotline, and the number of EVD suspect cases arriving at EHUs of their own volition, thereby helping policy makers assess and monitor the use and effectiveness of the national hotline.
- Maintain a database of all suspect EVD cases in the Western Area and their paths to testing and treatment, eventually enabling status updates to be given to families as required.

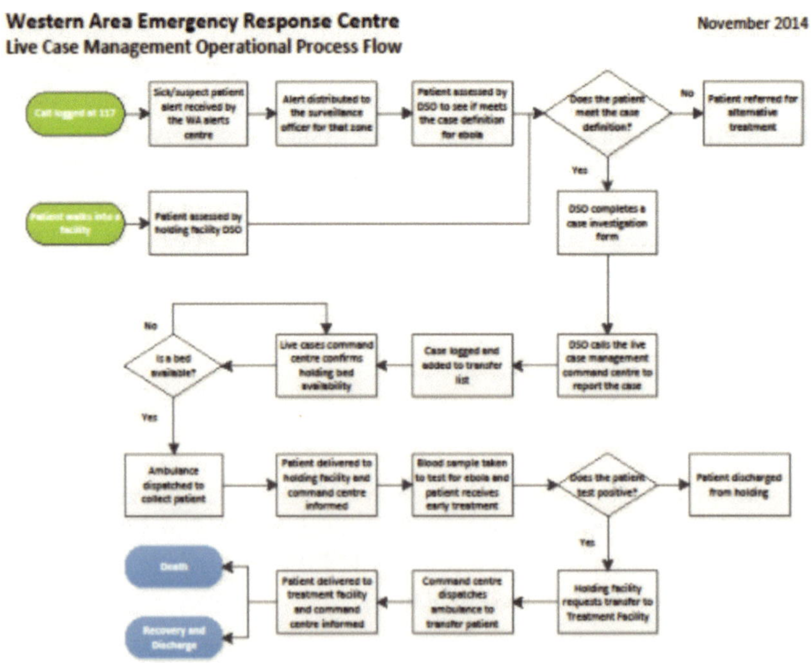

Figure 3. Live case management operational flow.

http://dx.doi.org/10.5772/63440

7.5.1. SMS Platform

KSLP supported an SMS platform to relay laboratory results to EHUs as close as possible to the publication of results. This was crucial in a low-resource setting with limited internet and data sharing capabilities, and the system was later adopted by laboratories in the Western Area. Relaying results via SMS from source sought to minimise errors in communication and create accountability for the reporting of results by creating a record of time between the receipt of results by the Live Case Management Command Cell and the time results were relayed by SMS.

7.6. Lasting capacity

By the time KSLP phased out its support of the Western Area DERC in March 2015, a team of twenty national volunteers were able to confidently manage the Live Case Management Cell, and continued to utilise the systems KSLP helped to put in place to manage case flow. A number of national staff were seconded during later periods of the outbreak to support and mentor teams in other districts of Sierra Leone.

8. Legacy of EVD partnership working

Moving forward, KSLP has ongoing partnership and collaboration with the national secretary of HIV and TB, providing technical support for training, elaboration and implementation of treatment and management guidelines. Together we have established the first infectious diseases unit in the country at the main referral hospital, and will work with the medical school to undertake teaching of medical students in infectious diseases.

KSLP will assist Connaught in creating a Centre of Excellence in Infectious diseases to be a hub for care, education and research of infectious diseases. The main aims are to build individual, institution and national clinical research capacity in infectious disease response, with a focus on three work streams:

- Human resources—training hospital staff and students to plan, lead, and undertake clinical research;
- Research infrastructure—establishing the necessary infrastructure to support clinical research activity;
- Enabling environment—creating an enabling environment for clinical research across both main adult hospitals in Freetown, as part of a national clinical research agenda.

There is also very limited information available on antimicrobial resistance across the region, and KSLP aims to work with Connaught and partners in developing protocols for clinical management of patients based on a variety of syndromic management. The new ID unit will have an electronic patient record established in order to track demographics and clinical syndromes of patients. Other areas of clinical activity will include the ongoing care of those suffering sequelae of EVD infection, as ongoing IPC and WASH developments continue. KSLP and Connaught are also working with MOHS to initiate free tertiary care for adult Ebola survivors at the hospital.

These outcomes described were delivered through a partnership model. In this chapter we have revisited the various stages of the EVD outbreak, from early triage and case definitions, through ramping up isolation and treatment capacity, to how best to retain and develop resilience in health systems, alongside research efforts and outbreak control principles. We hope we have highlighted how an embedded organisation working in close collaboration with senior leaders in an MOHS hospital and other partners can assist in developing institutional and national response.

Glossary

Central Medical Stores	CMS
College of Medicine & Allied Health Sciences	COMAHS
Community Care Centre	CCC
District Ebola Response Centre	DERC
District Health Management Team	DHMT
Disease Surveillance Officer	DSO
Ebola Holding Unit	EHU
Ebola Response Consortium	ERC
Ebola Treatment Centre	ETC
Ebola Virus Disease	EVD
Health Care Worker	HCW
Human Immunodeficiency Virus	HIV
Infection Prevention and Control	IPC
Key Performance Indicators	KPI
King's Health Partners	KHP
King's Sierra Leone Partnership	KSLP
National Ebola Response Centre	NERC
Non-Governmental Organisations	NGOs
Personal Protective Equipment	PPE
Polymerase chain reaction	PCR
Public Health England	PHE
Rapid Diagnostic Test	RDT
Tuberculosis	TB
Ministry of Health & Sanitation	MOHS
Water, sanitation & hygiene	WASH

http://dx.doi.org/10.5772/63440

Author details

King's Sierra Leone Partnership:

Colin S Brown[1,2*], Mohamed Elsherbiny[1], Oliver Johnson[1], Amardeep Kamboz[1], Marta Lado[1], Andrew Leather[1], Natalie Mounter[1], Suzanne Thomas[1], Dan Youkee[1], Naomi Walker[1,3]

Ministry of Health & Sanitation and Connaught Hospital:

Waheed Awonuga[4], TB Kamara[4,5], Cecilia Kamara[5], Quaanan Kessete[4], Ramatu Ngauja[5]

1 King's Sierra Leone Partnership, King's Centre for Global Health, King's College London, and King's Health Partners, London, United Kingdom

2 Hospital for Tropical Diseases, University College London Hospital, London, United Kingdom

3 Department of Clinical Research, London School of Hygiene and Tropical Medicine, London, United Kingdom

4 College of Medicine and Allied Health Sciences, Freetown, Sierra Leone

5 Ministry of Health and Sanitation, Sierra Leone

*Address all correspondence to: colin.1.brown@kcl.ac.uk

References

[1] Oxfam. Building Resilient Health Systems and Learning from the Ebola Crisis. Oxford: Oxfam, 2015.

[2] World Health Organization. World Health Statistics 2015. Geneva: WHO, 2015.

[3] WHO. Ebola Situation Summary: data as of 2nd March 2016. Geneva: WHO, 2016.

[4] Gonzalez JP, Pourrut X, Leroy E. Ebolavirus and other filoviruses. Current Topics in Microbiology and Immunology 2007;315:363–87.

[5] Pigott DM, Golding N, Mylne A, et al. Mapping the zoonotic niche of Ebola virus disease in Africa. eLife 2014;3:e04395.

[6] Gire SK, Goba A, Andersen KG, et al. Genomic surveillance elucidates Ebola virus origin and transmission during the 2014 outbreak. Science 2014;345:1369–72.

[7] Brown CS, Cropley I. Ebola virus disease: where are we now and where do we go. Postgrad Med J 2014;90:610–12.

[8] UK Government Press Release. First British Ebola treatment facility opens in Sierra Leone. London: Gov. UK, 2014.

[9] Olu O, Cormican M, Kamara KB, Butt W. Community Care Centre (CCC) as adjunct in the management of Ebola Virus Disease (EVD) cases during outbreaks: experience from Sierra Leone. Pan African Medical Journal 2015;22:Suppl 1–14.

[10] Brown CS, Arkell P, Rokadiya S. Ebola virus disease – the 'Black Swan' in West Africa. Tropical Doctor 2015;45(1):2–5.

[11] Johnson O, Youkee D, Brown CS, et al. Ebola Holding Units at Government Hospitals in Sierra Leone: evidence for a flexible and effective model for safe isolation, early treatment initiation, hospital safety, and health system functioning. BMJ Global Health, accepted for publication

[12] King's Sierra Leone Partnership. A Guide for the Establishment & Supervision of Ebola Holding Units. Freetown: KSLP, 2014.

[13] Boumandouki P, Formenty P, Epelboin A, et al. Clinical management of patients and deceased during the Ebola outbreak from October to December 2003 in Republic of Congo. Bulletin De La Societe De Pathologie Exotique 2005;98(3):218–23 [in French].

[14] Roddy P, Howard N, Van Kerkhove MD, et al. Clinical manifestations and case management of Ebola haemorrhagic fever caused by a newly identified virus strain, Bundibugyo, Uganda, 2007–2008. PLoS One 2012;7(12):e52986.

[15] Guimard Y, Bwaka MA, Colebunders R, et al. Organization of patient care during the Ebola hemorrhagic fever epidemic in Kikwit, Democratic Republic of the Congo, 1995. Journal of Infectious Diseases 1999;179 Suppl 1:S268–73.

[16] Nkoghe D, Kone ML, Yada A, Leroy E. A limited outbreak of Ebola haemorrhagic fever in Etoumbi, Republic of Congo, 2005. Transactions of the Royal Society of Tropical Medicine and Hygiene 2011;105(8):466–72.

[17] Lado M, Walker NF, Baker P, et al. Clinical features of patients isolated for suspected Ebola virus disease at Connaught Hospital, Freetown, Sierra Leone: a retrospective cohort study. Lancet ID 2015;15(9):1024–33.

[18] Brown CS, Kessete Q, Baker P, et al. Bottlenecks in health systems functioning for control of Ebola Virus Disease in Connaught Hospital, Freetown, Sierra Leone. Poster Presentation P0092, European Conference on Clinical Microbiology and Infectious Diseases, Amsterdam, 2016.

[19] Arkel P, Youkee D, Brown CS, et al. Quantifying the risk of nosocomial infection within Ebola Holding Units: a retrospective cohort study of negative patients discharged from

five Ebola Holding Units in Western Area, Sierra Leone. Tropical Medicine & International Health, March 2016, accepted pending minor revisions.

[20] Fitzpatrick G, Vogt F, Moi Gbabai OB, et al. Describing readmissions to an Ebola case management centre (CMC), Sierra Leone, 2014. Euro Surveillance 2014;19(40):pii=20924.

[21] Youkee D, Brown CS, Lilburn P. Assessment of environmental contamination and environmental decontamination practices within an ebola holding unit, Freetown, Sierra Leone. PLoS One 2015;DOI:10.1371/journal.pone.0145167.

[22] Walker NF, Brown CS, Youkee D, et al. Evaluation of a point-of-care blood test for identification of Ebola virus disease at Ebola holding units, Western Area, Sierra Leone, January to February 2015. Euro Surveillance 2015;20(12):pii=21073.

[23] Gibson T. An Extraordinary 19 Months. London: Royal College of Physicians, 2015. https://www.rcplondon.ac.uk/news/extraordinary-19-months.

[24] Connaught Hospital, unpublished data.

[25] Bundu I, Patel A, Mansaray A, Kamara TB, Hunt LM. Surgery in the time of Ebola: how events impacted on a single surgical institution in Sierra Leone. Journal of the Royal Army Medical Corps 2016;pii: jramc-2015-000582.

[26] Kingham TP, Kamara TB, Cherian MN, et al. Quantifying surgical capacity in Sierra Leone: a guide for improving surgical care. Archives of Surgery 2009;144(2):122–7.

[27] Youkee D, Williams N, Laggah M, et al. The impact of the 2014–15 Ebola virus disease epidemic on emergency care attendance and capacity at a tertiary referral hospital in Freetown, Sierra Leone: a retrospective observational study. Lancet 2016;387(S109):http://dx.doi.org/10.1016/S0140-6736(16)00496-7.

[28] Dunn AC, Walker TA, Redd J, et al. Nosocomial transmission of Ebola virus disease on pediatric and maternity wards: Bombali and Tonkolili, Sierra Leone, 2014. American Journal of Infection Control 2016;1;44(3):269–72.

[29] Borchert M, Mutyaba I, Van Kerkhove MD, et al. Ebola haemorrhagic fever outbreak in Masindi District, Uganda: outbreak description and lessons learned. BMC Infectious Diseases 2011;11:357.

[30] Fisher-Hoch SP. Lessons from nosocomial viral haemorrhagic fever outbreaks. British Medial Bulletin 2005;73–74:123–37.

[31] Baron RC, McCormick JB, Zubeir OA. Ebola virus disease in southern Sudan: hospital dissemination and intrafamilial spread. Bulletin of the World Health Organisation 1983;61(6):997–1003.

[32] Kilmarx PH, Clarke KR, Dietz PM, et al. Ebola virus disease in health care workers? Sierra Leone, 2014. Morbidity & Mortality Weekly Report 2014;63(49):1168–71.

Chapter 3

Ebola Preparedness and Risk in Latin America

Alfonso J. Rodriguez-Morales,
Jaime Andrés Cardona-Ospina,
Sivia Fernanda-Urbano,
Katherinn Melissa Nasner-Posso,
Stefania Cruz-Calderón,
Carlos E. Calvache-Benavides,
Yudy Lorena Delgado-Pascuaza,
Juan Camilo Castillo, Maria Yamile Alvarez-Ríos,
Hamilton A. Marín-Rincón, Liceth Urrutia and
Alberto Paniz-Mondolfi

Additional information is available at the end of the chapter

http://dx.doi.org/10.5772/62945

Abstract

Until today, February 22, 2016, no confirmed Ebola cases have been diagnosed in Americas (except USA, four cases with one death). Confusion, lack of knowledge, and fear have led to quickly misclassify cases as suspected, when in fact most of them are false alarms. Nevertheless, European governments summoned to mobilize resources to attend the Ebola outbreak in West Africa. And also Latin American governments should contribute to halt this humanitarian crisis and to be prepared for the potential arrival of this deadly virus in the Caribbean, Central, and South American mainland. In this chapter, we described the experience of preparedness as well as risk assessment done in Latin America regarding the threat of Ebola for the region.

Keywords: Ebola, preparedness, risk assessment, travel medicine, Latin America

1. Introduction

Ebola virus (EBOV) was the second genus of the Filoviridae family to be discovered. This negative-sense, single-stranded RNA virus was first identified in 1976 following two simultaneous outbreaks in Zaïre (now known as the Democratic Republic of Congo) and Sudan [1–4]. Since then, at least 25 subsequent outbreaks, including the ongoing outbreak in West Africa, have occurred and various EBOV species have been identified with genetic and virulence variability and still unknown pathogenesis. Before 2014, none of those epidemics implied imported cases outside Africa, with its multiple implications [1–9].

Nowadays, the ongoing outbreak (almost finished) in West Africa has been the largest reported in history, and from a global health perspective, it showed again how poverty, cultural practices, and weak and unprepared health systems could interact exacerbating infectious disease spread, limiting its control and mitigation, and the importance of travel in a globalized world, since this was the first outbreak in which EBOV cases and transmission were reported outside of Africa [5, 6, 8].

This outbreak has challenged global capability of response of world policymakers to organize and implement resources in an impoverished and previous overlooked area, it taught the implication of reactive rather than proactive health systems organization, and in a setting of unpreparedness and lack of knowledge, social media played an important role in spreading unfounded fear through false alarms [5, 6, 8].

Until today, February 14, 2016, a total of 28,639 cases and 11,316 deaths (case fatality rate [CFR %] of 39.5%) were reported according to the World Health Organization (WHO) report of February 17, 2016 [10]. The majority of these cases and deaths occurred between August and December 2014, after which case incidence declined apparently associated with scale-up of treatment, isolation, and safe burial.

In the last 21 days, zero cases were reported in the implicated countries (Guinea, Liberia, and Sierra Leone) and on November 7, 2015, December 29, 2015, and January 14, 2016, the WHO declared that human-to-human transmission of Ebola virus has ended in Guinea, Sierra Leone, and Liberia, respectively, if no further cases appear, entering in a period of heightened surveillance, putting these countries in the way on recovery, and giving the chance of getting essential health services backup and to address weaknesses to rebuild a resilient health system [10].

Likewise, there were a total of seven cases reported outside of African continent with one death at USA [10]. Countries involving imported cases outside Africa have been Italy, Spain, United Kingdom, and USA (each one with one case, except USA with four cases) [11] (**Figure 1**), without truly suspected cases in Latin America and the Caribbean (LAC) [6–13].

Nevertheless, European governments summoned to mobilize resources to attend the Ebola outbreak in West Africa during the peak of the epidemics [14–16]. But also LAC governments have been called to contribute to halt this humanitarian crisis and to be prepared for the potential arrival of this deadly virus in the Caribbean, Central, and South American mainland, particularly during the peak of the epidemics in Africa. In this chapter, we described the experience of risk assessment as well as preparedness done in Latin America regarding the threat of Ebola for the region.

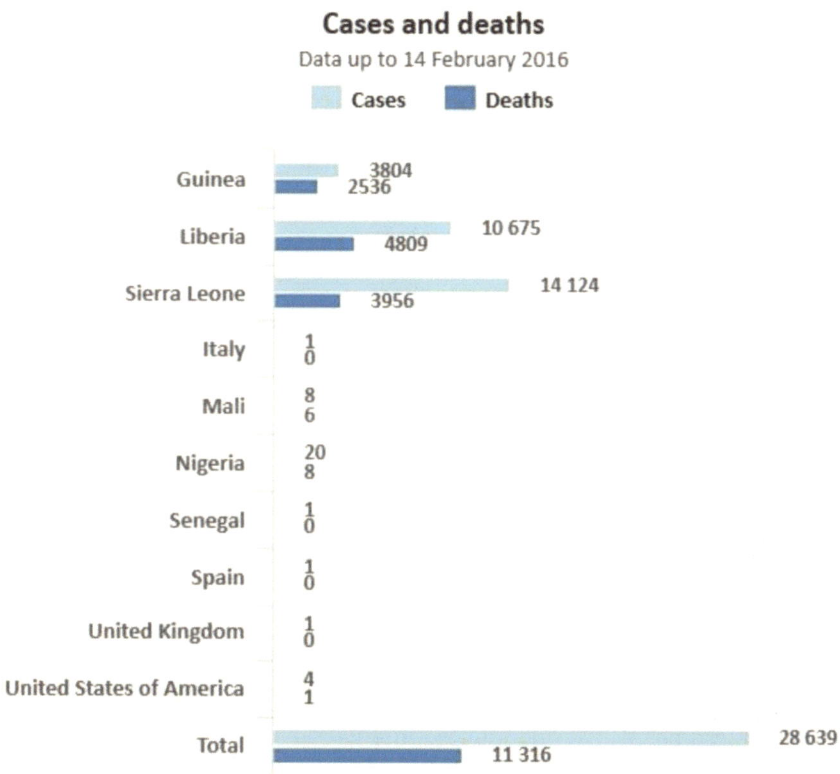

Figure 1. Confirmed, probable, and suspected EVD cases worldwide. From: WHO Ebola Situation Report – February 17, 2016.

2. Risk assessment

Some studies have provided perspectives on the potential for Ebola virus disease (EVD) to spread across international borders via commercial air travel [17–20]. However, they have only focused on top international destinations in Africa, Europe, Asia, and North America. Recently, we have assessed this for Latin American countries.

During the peak of the epidemics, we gathered epidemiological data from the Ebola response roadmap situation report of the World Health Organization (WHO) (for October 29, 2014) [20]. We included Sierra Leone, Guinea, and Liberia as officially affected regions by the EVD epidemics. Because data concerning commercial air travel out of Guinea, Liberia, and Sierra

Leone to LAC countries were unavailable, we used population migration data from the United Nations' international migrant stock by destination and origin database (estimates of the international migrant stock exodus for the midpoint [1 July] of each year: 1990, 2000, 2010, and 2013). We assessed the number of people migrating from Guinea, Liberia, and Sierra Leone to LAC countries in years 2000, 2010, and 2013. We also included within those numbers all potential returns of previously deployed persons from LAC countries to affected West African nations. We took the maximum number of migrating people from West African countries to LAC during those three years, as the potential number of people migrating in 2014, followed by an estimation on the prevalence of EBV in source countries (cases/100,000 pop and %), based on WHO reports and official population estimates, gathered from the World Bank registry data. We assumed a random distribution of prevalence among population as equal for migrating people in order to calculate the number of potential persons migrating with EBV to CSA countries [8].

Up to October 29, 2014, WHO reported 13,676 cases of EBV, with 6535 cases from Liberia, Sierra Leone (5235), and Guinea (1906). During the last 21 days, 1433 active cases were reported in Sierra Leone, 867 in Liberia, and 666 in Guinea, revealing prevalence rates for this period of 23.52 cases/100,000 pop (0.0235%), 20.19 cases/100,000 pop (0.0202%), and 5.67 cases/100,000 pop (0.0057%), respectively [8, 20].

Based on those prevalence rates and assuming migration numbers would be similar for 2014, we estimated the potential number of people with EVD relying on each country's individual prevalence, which resulted in a probability of less than 1 possible EVD case potentially arriving to LAC countries. Assuming the same prevalence of active cases, migration should increase up to 4255 persons/year from Sierra Leone, 4950 from Liberia, and 17,544 from Guinea, to reach at least 1 case in some Latin American countries [8].

Previous reports estimated that one infected international air traveler would leave Guinea every 2.7 months, Liberia every 0.2 months, and Sierra Leone every 0.6 months [17–20]. However, such numbers may represent an underestimate of the real situation if we take into consideration the fact of potential cases originating from the shipping sector and spreading through maritime transport. In addition, connection flights (e.g. Bogota, Colombia to Monrovia, and Liberia with connections at New York, USA, and Casablanca, Morocco) may increase the odds of affected passengers to reach Latin America from these countries by connecting through such alternate bridging destinations [8].

Based on the aforementioned facts, the possibility of EVD spreading to Latin America raises concerns in regard to the capacity of healthcare institutions and laboratories in the region to provide adequate facilities, competently trained healthcare staff, acceptable infection control measures and equipment, supplies, protocols and resources to provide effective disease management, diagnosis, and overall containment strategies [6, 8]. Previously, WHO published the public health actions for early detection and prevention of transmission of Ebola and Marburg viruses. Even in a low-risk setting, there are significant concerns over whether Latin American countries are ready to face EVD within their vulnerable healthcare systems [6, 8]. Fortunately, after the epidemics in Africa, none confirmed cases nor real suspected cases arrived to Latin America, although most countries in the region, particularly Brazil and

Colombia, were prepared for the arrival, developed national guidelines for preparedness, and managed some false alarms properly, in most of the cases.

3. Preparedness

We acknowledged a huge need for field-based laboratories, epidemiological and microbiological surveillance resources, diagnostic equipment, and mobile communications software as well as other technological assets. As revealed by the ongoing chikungunya and Zika epidemics [21–25], LAC is particularly vulnerable to infectious disease spreading given that there is a lack of appropriate healthcare infrastructure to tackle a challenge of such dimensions, particularly from airborne (e.g. Influenza H1N1 in 2009) and vector-borne diseases [22, 26]. However, regarding the collaboration to intervene the crisis, it is important to highlight that the Cuban government sent a team of 165 highly trained healthcare professionals to assist and mitigate the epidemic, being, so far, the largest medical team that any single foreign country sent out to the field, from LAC to Africa [6, 8].

Besides that, the Pan American Health Organization (PAHO) [15], along with the WHO, have recommended nations to implement measures based on surveillance [20], laboratory diagnosis, case management, infection prevention and control, clinical management and awareness and communication. This in order to be prepared and to have an appropriate response to the hypothetical arrival of EVD to LAC, which as has been mentioned, was expected to be low to very low [6, 8]. Although early detection, tracing, and isolation of truly suspected cases and contacts would limit the risk of disease spread, the proper laboratory assessment and sample management will be restricted given the lack of trained health personnel, protective equipment, and adequate transport particularly in some highly densely populated areas, where poverty and deficient basic services constitute a melting point for the development of potential outbreaks. Health personnel must be capable to manage risk group 4 pathogen, as EBOV, and must account with protective equipment like non-sterile gloves, masks, goggles preferably with an anti-fog visor and apron or waterproof apron, disposable if possible [6, 8, 16, 18]. Additionally, staff in charge of handling and transporting the samples must account with a certification by the International Air Transport Association for shipping and handling Category A infectious substance in order to send samples to the only two laboratories in the region that can receive them: the National Center for Emerging Zoonotic Infectious Diseases (NCEZID), Centers for Disease Control and Prevention (CDC) and Zoonotic Diseases and Special Pathogens, National Microbiology Laboratory, Infectious Disease and Emergency Preparedness Branch Public Health Agency of Canada. Furthermore, as opposed to Europe, where BSL-4 (BSL-4) laboratories network already exists, LAC still requires a significant increase in technical partnership as well as other resource capabilities, BSL-4 in LAC are scarce what has limited the work with other important BSL-4 required viral pathogens endemic to the region, such as hantaviruses in the past and in the middle of current of cases of this zoonotic viruses in Chile and other countries in the region [6, 8, 16, 18].

On the other hand, if EBOV arrives to LAC, it would pose an immense diagnostic challenge in a region where endemic viral hemorrhagic fevers exhibit remarkable similar clinical findings. Distinguishing cases of Guanarito (Venezuela), Machupo (Bolivia), Junín (Argentina), and Sabiá (Brazil) viruses from Ebola, as well as from other highly prevalent infections such as yellow fever, dengue with hemorrhagic manifestations, leptospirosis, and typhoid fever, among others, will constitute an ever-increasing challenge. Point-of-care testing using a biothreat panel like the BioFire diagnostics BioSurveillance system would be useful for screening highly suspicious cases, while at the same time, providing an automated sample-to-answer diagnostic platform in areas with lack of healthcare trained personnel, even though rapid diagnostic test use is discouraged given its low specificity. We still do not know how such tests would perform in a non-prevalent Ebola region, and at the same time, it could be cost prohibitive for many governments in the hemisphere [6, 8, 16, 18].

Otherwise, the clinical management of those suspected and confirmed cases should be at designated hospitals that must comply with contact isolation conditions, ideally individually and not by cohorts of suspected or confirmed cases, appropriate provisions of personal protective equipment, and health services with personnel trained in infection prevention and control [6, 8, 16, 18]. These characteristics probably are lacking even in some intermediate cities of LAC forcing to translate patients to places where these are attained and making to consider that transport of those patients needs special protective measures too. Even more, healthcare institutions should start joining efforts to design preparedness and response programs in order to revamp or build up de novo infrastructure to properly address suspicious cases and prepare healthcare professionals for caring of confirmed Ebola-infected patients. It is also important to coordinate this LAC response to Ebola with the guidance of the regional multilateral health organisms: The PAHO should lead this process; and the recently created South American Institute of Government in Health (www.isags-unasur.org) and the South American National Institutes of Health Network could demonstrate their ability to recruit and materialize resources for global health [6, 8, 16, 18].

The call for attention that was the EBOV outbreak highlighted the importance of proactive organization of health systems particularly in those settings in which poverty, social inequality, and lack of basic healthcare services and facilities could limit action when an infectious disease has established [6, 8, 16, 18]. Many countries in LAC have proved its restraints in infectious disease control, as recently reported for malaria, dengue, chikungunya, and Zika in Venezuela, and its social and economic context can act as boosters for infection spread [22, 26]. As taught, the entire world needs to turn out its look and watch for those impoverished areas before crisis, searching to close gaps in order to reach fairer societies.

Latin America is endemic for many febrile infectious diseases conditions; then, signs and symptoms of EVD may overlap with other acute viral hemorrhagic fevers like dengue, chikungunya, and now Zika posing a challenge at the time of diagnosis [9]. Despite the low-risk for a local outbreak in LAC, the possibility of an imported case always remains latent [6, 8]. Thus, in light of such hypothetical epidemiological scenario, we also considered that assessing knowledge and perceptions among healthcare students and workers about the epidemiology, transmission, and clinical manifestations of Ebola in a country like Colombia is of utmost importance; particularly, taking into account that before the 2014–2015 epidemic, no information concerning EVD was available in Colombia's public health surveillance program [9]. Then, an observational, descriptive, cross-sectional study was conducted among 107 healthcare workers attending the symposium "What we should know about Ebola?" (organized by the Coffee Triangle regional chapter of the Colombian Association of Infectious Diseases and the Universidad Tecnológica de Pereira) held in October (2014) in one city of Colombia: Pereira, Risaralda [9]. Attendees who agreed to be part of the research (convenience sample) filled out a basic knowledge questionnaire, which included aspects on the epidemiology, symptoms, and prevention of the disease (five questions). Questionnaires were completed before and after the event. Statistical analysis was performed using the SPSS statistical package, version 19.0. A chi-square test ($p < 0.05$) was run to assess the significance and compare observed frequencies of correct answers before and after the symposium. The results obtained for each individual question revealed an increasing statistical significance when comparing presurvey to postsurvey answers ($p < 0.05$), highlighting the pivotal role of disease prevention, surveillance, preparedness, and response informational resources [9].

As healthcare workers, it is essential to rely on complete and updated information about emergent diseases such as EVD, a disease which has recently been cataloged by WHO as an international public health emergency. Unfortunately, to date, many aspects on the basic ecology, transmission, and pathogenesis of the disease remain unclear. The possibility that different species of bats and primates endemic to the New World could serve as hosts for the virus remains a lurking possibility, as well as a threat to the possible arrival of this disease to the Americas [9].

A lack of experience on how to recognize its signs and symptoms as well as how to approach and manage outbreaks still remains a challenge in most affected countries and a most inherent peril to unaffected regions. All in all, it is imperative to call for awareness and prepare to handle and recognize this disease, for which world class organizations like the CDC and WHO have already issued the necessary guidelines on how to prevent possible epidemics through early recognition of cases, as well as how to achieve prompt institution of containment measures [9].

Due to a lack of efficient healthcare policies and systems, Latin American countries are particularly vulnerable to infectious diseases, as it has been shown with other endemic infectious maladies such as chikungunya, Zika, and malaria [22–26]. In view of this, besides preparing for preventive and interventional actions, educational resources should also aim to battle the negative impact of misinformation and fear, which may lead to jitters as a consequence of false alarm cases which occurred in fact in LAC in the middle of the epidemics of EVD in Africa [6–9].

Informational and educational tools play on improving knowledge about clinical manifestations and disease management among caregivers residing in non-affected areas, as well as how to respond if challenged to face such an unlikely event, in this case, in LAC [9].

4. False alarms

During the epidemics of Ebola in Africa and the arrival of imported cases to Europe and North America, fear and alert were combined in LAC regarding the potential arrival of suspected cases of EVD in this region [6–9]. As consequence of that, confusion, lack of knowledge, and fear led to quickly misclassify cases as suspected, when in fact most of them are false alarms. Latin America was challenged with false alarms of "suspected" cases of EVD that not met the criteria to be classified as real suspected cases.

Our group assessed false alarms and suspected cases in the Americas of EVD, based on online available information on such cases. Analyzing online news information sources, data on suspected cases were collected and the WHO Ebola fever suspected case definition reviewed in order to classify them as suspected or false alarms.

Until April 1, 2015, 67 reports, containing 232 suspected or false alarm cases, were retrieved from the Web in 25 American countries. From them, 79.1% corresponded to false alarms and 20.9% suspected cases (WHO complied definition). From false alarms, only 18.9% came from Sierra Leone (13%), Liberia (4%), or Guinea (2%), but none of them presented symptoms during last 21 days (**Figure 2**). Although those cases not met the definitions, were considered suspected cases and then reported as that. From real suspected cases (14), all came from Ebola endemic places (28.6% Nigeria, 21.4% Guinea, 7.1% Liberia, 7.1% Sierra Leona), all of them with symptoms (mostly fever) during the last 21 days (**Figure 3**).

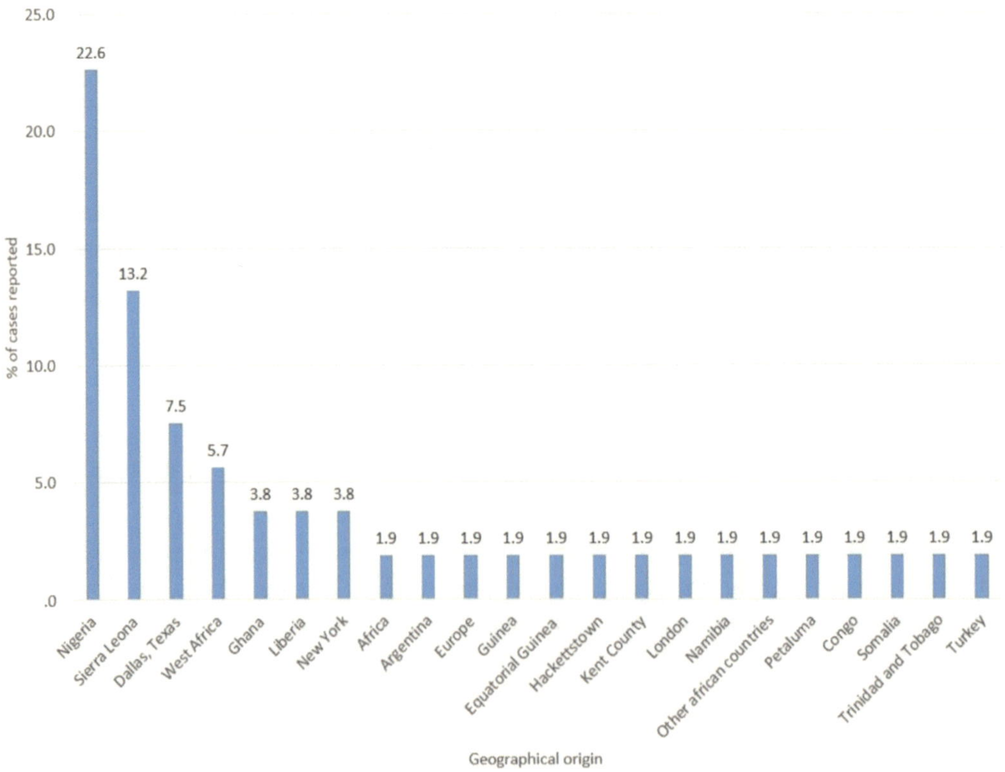

Figure 2. Geographical origin of the false alarm cases.

http://dx.doi.org/10.5772/62945

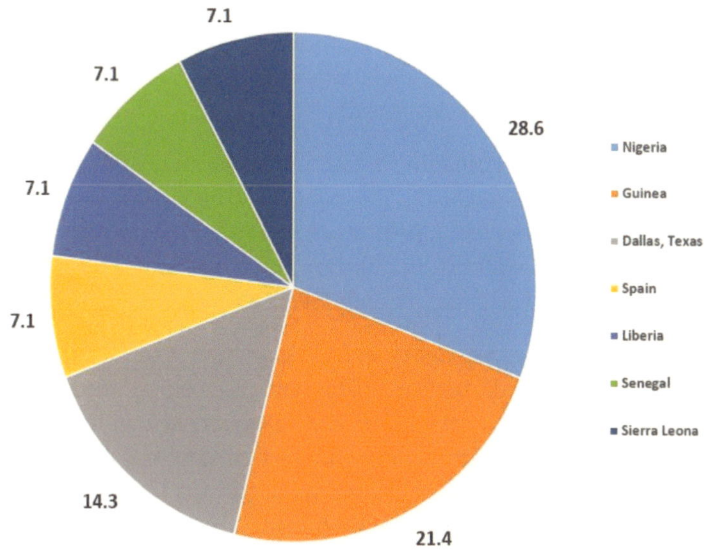

Figure 3. Geographical origin of the suspected cases (met WHO definition of suspected case).

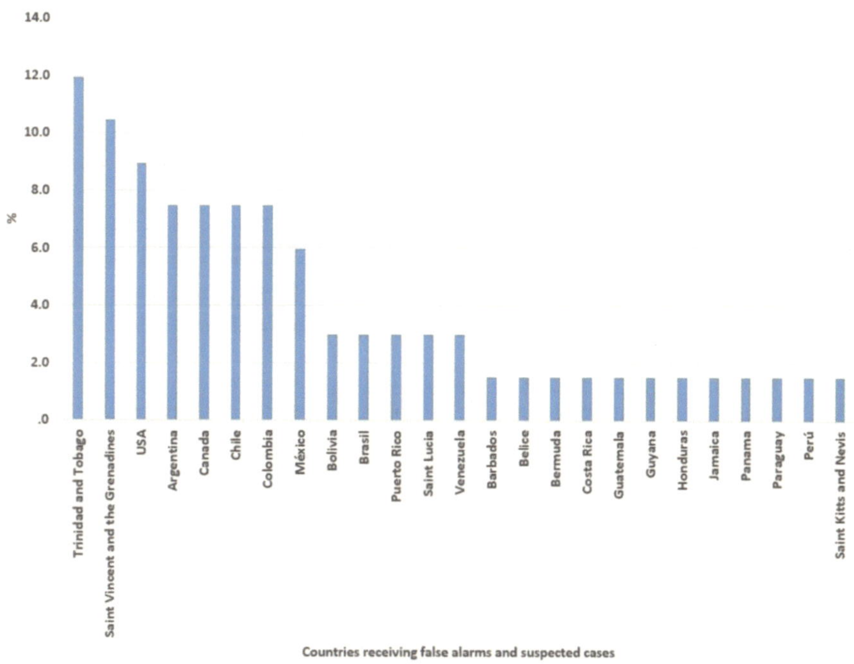

Figure 4. Countries receiving false alarms and suspected cases.

With regard to the countries receiving these cases (suspected and false alarms), most corresponded to Trinidad and Tobago (11.9%), followed by Saint Vincent and the Grenadines

(10.4%), USA (9.0%), Argentina (7.5%), Canada (7.5%), Chile (7.5%), Colombia (7.5%), and Mexico (6.0%) (**Figure 4**). These findings were consistent with the risk assessment previously performed based on the migration and travel patterns from EVD risk countries from Africa to potential countries in LAC region, as described.

Although the possibility of Ebola spreading to Latin America always has been low, as previous models have shown, concerns in regard to the capacity of healthcare institutions and laboratories in the region are real. Even more, healthcare workers in the region are not prepared at all. Then, actions include reinforcement of infection control actions in healthcare settings and access to high-quality diagnosis testing, among others, should be enhanced.

The world experienced the largest epidemic of EVD known in extension and duration to date, since the virus was first identified back in 1976, with cases being reported beyond African borders [1–10, 20]. There was, as a consequence, a sharp increase in the number of research and publications related to vaccine candidates and the immunological aspects of EVD, among other aspects [1, 6, 8]. Although not particularly affected by a large number of cases in this current outbreak, the United States has played historically and continues to play on Ebola research, although other countries have also contributed. Also, cooperation played a key role among different nations, particularly between African, European, and North American countries, but this should be enhanced for future epidemics as already occurred in 2014, considering also the possibility in the future of suspected cases in Latin America and the Caribbean [1, 16].

Author details

Alfonso J. Rodriguez-Morales[1,2,3*], Jaime Andrés Cardona-Ospina[1], Sivia Fernanda-Urbano[1], Katherinn Melissa Nasner-Posso[1], Stefania Cruz-Calderón[1], Carlos E. Calvache-Benavides[1], Yudy Lorena Delgado-Pascuaza[1], Juan Camilo Castillo[1], Maria Yamile Alvarez-Ríos[1], Hamilton A. Marín-Rincón[1], Liceth Urrutia[1] and Alberto Paniz-Mondolfi[2,3,4]

*Address all correspondence to: arodriguezm@utp.edu.co

1 Public Health and Infection Research Group, Faculty of Health Sciences, Technological University of Pereira, Pereira, Risaralda, Colombia

2 Working Group on Zoonoses, International Society for Chemotherapy, Aberdeen, United Kingdom

3 Committee on Travel Medicine, Pan-American Association of Infectious Diseases, Quito, Ecuador

4 Department of Pathology and Laboratory Medicine, International Hospital, Barquisimeto, Venezuela and the Laboratory of Biochemistry, Institute of Biomedicine/Venezuelan Institute of Social Security (IVSS), Caracas, Venezuela

References

[1] Cruz-Calderón S, Nasner-Posso KM, Alfaro-Toloza P, Paniz-Mondolfi AE, Rodríguez-Morales AJ. A bibliometric analysis of global Ebola research. Travel Medicine and Infectious Disease. 2015 March–April;13(2):202–4.

[2] Fazekas B, Fazekas J, Moledina M, Fazekas B, Karolyhazy K Ebola virus disease: awareness among junior doctors in England. The Journal of Hospital Infection. 2015. Jul;90(3):260–2. doi:10.1016/j.jhin.2015.03.007.

[3] Olival KJ, Hayman DT Filoviruses in bats: current knowledge and future directions. Viruses. 2014;6:1759–88.

[4] Peters CJ. Marburg and Ebola virus hemorrhagic fevers. In: Mandell GM, Douglas RG, Bennett JE (Eds.). Principles and practice of infectious diseases. New York: Churchill Livingstone. 2010;2259–63.

[5] Cardona-Ospina JA, Giselle-Badillo A, Calvache-Benavides CE, Rodriguez-Morales AJ. Ebola virus disease: an emerging zoonosis with importance for travel medicine. Travel Medicine and Infectious Disease. 2014;12:682–3.

[6] Rodriguez-Morales AJ, Henao DE, Franco TB, Mayta-Tristan P, Alfaro-Toloza P, Paniz-Mondolfi AE. Ebola: a latent threat to Latin America. Are we ready? Travel Medicine and Infectious Disease. 2014;12:688–9.

[7] Organization WHO. Ebola virus disease - Fact sheet. 2014. http://www.who.int/mediacentre/factsheets/fs103/en/

[8] Rodriguez-Morales AJ, Marin-Rincon HA, Sepulveda-Arias JC, Paniz-Mondolfi AE Assessing the potential migration of people from Ebola affected West African countries to Latin America. Travel Medicine and Infectious Disease. 2015. May–Jun;13(3):264–6. doi:10.1016/j.tmaid.2014.12.015.

[9] Patiño-Barbosa AM, Arroyave-Valencia F, García-Ramírez LM, Vallejo-Atehortúa E, Arciniegas-Pantoja M, Rodriguez-Morales AJ, Paniz-Mondolfi AE. Healthcare students and workers' knowledge about epidemiology and symptoms of Ebola in one city of Colombia. Journal of Hospital Infection. 2015 August;90(4):356–8.

[10] WHO. Ebola Situation Reports. Available at http://apps.who.int/ebola/ebola-situation-reports (Accessed: February 22, 2016).

[11] Chevalier MS, Chung W, Smith J, Weil LM, Hughes SM, Joyner SN, et al. Ebola virus disease cluster in the United States--Dallas County, Texas, 2014. MMWR Morbidity and Mortality Weekly Report. 2014;63:1087–8.

[12] Rodriguez-Morales AJ, Castañeda-Hernández DM, McGregor A. What makes people talk about Ebola on social media? A retrospective analysis of Twitter use. Travel Medicine and Infectious Disease 2015;13(1):100–1.

[13] Henao DE, Abella-Marquez LM, Failoc-Rojas VE, Lagos-Grisales GJ, Rodríguez-Morales AJ. In the current context of emerging infectious diseases, it should join the global health teaching in medical programs in Latin America? Salud Pública de México. 2015 July–August;57(4):296–7.

[14] de La Vega MA, Stein D, Kobinger GP. Ebolavirus evolution: past and present. PLoS Pathogens. 2015;11(11):e1005221.

[15] Pan American Health Organization/World Health Organization. Preparedness and Response for introduction of Ebola virus disease (EVD) in the Americas 2014.

[16] Ter Meulen J. Priorities for research on tropical viruses after the 2014 Ebola epidemic. Journal of Clinical Virology 2014. J Clin Virol. 2015 Mar;64:107–8. doi:10.1016/j.jcv.2014.12.008.

[17] Bogoch II, Creatore MI, Cetron MS, Brownstein JS, Pesik N, Miniota J, et al. Assessment of the potential for international dissemination of Ebola virus via commercial air travel during the 2014 west African outbreak. The Lancet. 2015 Jan 3;385(9962):29–35. doi: 10.1016/S0140-6736(14)61828-6.

[18] Chen T, Ka-Kit Leung R, Liu R, Chen F, Zhang X, Zhao J, et al. Risk of imported Ebola virus disease in China. Travel Medicine and Infectious Disease 2014;12(6PA):650–658.

[19] Gomes MFC, Pastore y Piontti A, Rossi L, Chao D, Longini I, Halloran ME, et al. Assessing the international spreading risk associated with the 2014 West African Ebola outbreak. PLOS Currents Outbreaks. 2014. Available at http://currents.plos.org/outbreaks/article/assessing-the-international-spreading-risk-associated-with-the-2014-west-african-ebola-outbreak/ (Accessed: November 9, 2014).

[20] World Health Organization. Ebola and Marburg virus disease epidemics: preparedness, alert, control, and evaluation. Interim version 1.2, August 2014. Geneva: World Health Organization, 2014. Available at http://apps.who.int/iris/bitstream/10665/130160/1/WHO_HSE_PED_CED_2014.05_eng.pdf?ua=1&ua=1 (Accessed: November 5, 2014).

[21] Clouet-Huerta D, Alfaro-Toloza P, Rodriguez-Morales AJ. Chikungunya in the Americas: preparedness, surveillance and alert in Chile. Revista chilena de infectología 2014;31(6):761–2.

[22] Rodríguez-Morales AJ, Paniz-Mondolfi AE. Venezuela: far from the path to dengue and chikungunya control. Journal of Clinical Virology 2015 May;66:60–1.

[23] Alfaro-Toloza P, Clouet-Huerta DE, Rodríguez-Morales AJ. Chikungunya, the emerging migratory rheumatism. Lancet ID 2015 May;15(5):510–2.

[24] Rodriguez-Morales AJ. Dengue and chikungunya were not enough: now also Zika arrived, 2015 April–June;11(2):e3.

[25] Rodríguez-Morales AJ. Zika: the new arbovirus threat for Latin America. The Journal of Infection in Developing Countries 2015 June;9(6):684–5.

[26] Rodríguez-Morales AJ, Paniz-Mondolfi AE. Venezuela's failure in malaria control. The Lancet 2014 August 23;384(9944):663–4.

Section 2

Phylogenetic Analysis of Ebola Virus

Chapter 4

A Genomic Landscape of Haplotype Diversity and Signatures of Phylogeographic Distribution in Zaire Ebolavirus during the 2014 EVD Epidemic

Yue Teng, Yan Yu, Yuan Jin, Xiaoping An and Dan Feng

Additional information is available at the end of the chapter

http://dx.doi.org/10.5772/63247

Abstract

The Ebola virus (EBOV) disease epidemic from 2013 to 2015 is the largest in history, affecting multiple countries in West Africa. Genome sequencing of EBOV has revealed extensive genetic variation and mutation rate. The evolution and the variations among genotypes of EBOV observed remain low, which suggests that the viral haplotypes may be common in this transmission. To address this hypothesis, we investigated the genomic portrait of haplotype diversity in EBOV from 1976 to the 2014 outbreaks. We obtained 176 haplotypes in 305 gene-coding sequences of EBOV and found that the Hap8 in multiple viral haplotypes is the major epidemic lineage in the 2014 Sierra Leone outbreak. The phylogeographic analysis of EBOV transmission in Sierra Leone during 2014 outbreaks indicated that the genetic flow in EBOV was no more likely to occur within or without populations and the correlation between genetic and geographical distance is not significant. Our study first detected the diversity of viral haplotypes with systematic calculation of phylogeographic distribution in EBOV. This observation highlighted how Ebola virus is substantially different in virulence or transmissibility in comparison to the virus lineages associated with 2014 outbreaks in Sierra Leone, which provides a clue to understand the 2014 EBOV spreading.

Keywords: Ebolavirus, Genome sequencing, Evolutionary, Haplotype diversity, Phylogeographic distribution

1. Introduction

The recent Zaire Ebolavirus (EBOV) epidemic (2013–2015) was the largest in history, affecting multiple countries in West Africa.

The Zaire Ebolavirus (EBOV) is an unprecedented epidemic in West Africa during 2013 to 2015. Started from December 2013 in Guinea [1], the current EBOV outbreak spread into Liberia in March, into Sierra Leone in May, into Nigeria in late July, into Senegal in late August, and into Democratic Republic of Congo in early September [2]. Ebola virus disease (EVD) has become a global concern in 2014.

Genome sequencing of EBOV samples isolated from affected individuals during this outbreak revealed extensive viral genetic variation and mutations.

As the Ebola epidemic sweeps through West Africa, the genetic data of EBOV will answer some questions regarding the evolution dynamic of EBOV. Recently, *Tong et al.* published 175 genomes of EBOV [3], collected in Sierra Leone from September to November 2014 and *Hoene et al.* reported 4 viral genomes obtained in Mali from October to November 2014 [4]. Gire *et al.* published 99 genomes from 78 patients infected in or around Kenema, Sierra Leone during May and June of 2014 [5]. Additionally, Baize *et al.* released three EBOV genomes, collected in Guinea during March 2014 [1]. Those previous studies indicated that the EBOV is evolving slowly and is not undergoing rapid evolution in humans during the current outbreak [3, 4]. However, the detailed information of the lineage of virus, the viral mutational pattern, and the dispersal route among districts are still largely unknown, which should show the signatures of transmission and is of strategic importance to find the acquiring mutations evading diagnostic tests or vaccines [6–8].

Recent studies have investigated the genomic 'portrait' of haplotype diversity in EBOV outbreaks from 1976 onwards, and the recent major outbreak presented a unique opportunity to understand genetic variation and evolution with regards to EBOV.

Currently, the patterns of EBOV genomes variation within and between hosts have shown that human-to-human transmission can involve two or more viral haplotypes. It is possible to use geographic, temporal, and epidemiological metadata work together with the transmission clustering inferred from viral genetic data. Thus, we use the coding sequences of EBOV genomes from 1976 to 2014 to investigate haplotypes of EBOV and apply phylogeographic analysis on them [1, 3–5].

The aim of this chapter is to describe the methodology for the investigation of the genomic landscape of haplotype diversity and signatures of phylogeographic distribution in Ebola virus.

This study aims to identify the major haplotype of EBOV and the snapshot of transmission with viral genetic distance during this outbreak, which may shed light on the underlying mechanisms of EBOV spreading with a clear landscape of the 2014 outbreak.

2. Methods of investigating EBOV genetic differences

The diversity of viral haplotypes can be systematically calculated using a phylogeographic distribution approach. The following techniques that are required to understand the genetics of a viral outbreak will be described.

2.1. Sequencing

We obtained the available full-length genome sequences of EBOV, resulting 305 whole genomic sequences in total at this study, from Ebolavirus Resource in NCBI (http://www.ncbi.nlm.nih.gov/genome/viruses/variation/ebola/). The analysed EBOV genomes included 19 EBOV genomes from previous outbreaks before 2014, 99 genomes from Sierra Leone from May to June 2014, 6 sequences from Guinea in March 2014, 4 sequences from Mali 2014, 1 from Liberia in 2014, 1 from United Kingdom in 2014 and 175 newly viral genomic data during 25 September to 11 November from Sierra Leone. The sequences of EBOV-coding gene (NP, VP35, VP40, GP, VP30, VP24, L) were aligned using MAFFT v7.05.

2.2. Phylogenetic tree reconstruction

Phylogenetic trees were constructed with MrBayes v3.2 under the GTR model of nucleotide substitution and gamma-distributed rates among sites for 10 million generations. We sampled every 1000 steps and the first 25% of the samples were removed as burn-in. The convergence was checked when average standard deviation of split frequency was below 0.01 and all potential scale reduction factor (PSRF values approached 1.00). We also inferred maximum likelihood phylogenies (1000 bootstrap replicates) of EBOV under GTR+gamma model using RAxML v8.1.6.

2.3. Root-to-tip distance estimation

Root-to-tip distance of the 2014 EBOV was estimated using Path-O-Gen v1.4. The maximum likelihood tree inferred in the previous step was used as the input tree file and the root was placed on the common ancestral branch of Guinea isolates. The estimated root-to-tip divergence of each sample and the corresponding isolation date were projected to the same coordinate system.

2.4. Population analyses of haplotype networks based on specific towns or geographical distances

The populations were defined based on the town and geographical distances manually. The two towns within 40 km were considered as one population. DnaSP v.5.10.01 was used to generate haplotype data files and to calculate haplotype and nucleotide diversity for each population. The NETWORK software v.4.6.1.3 served to create a haplotype network using median-joining method. Population structure was assessed by calculating pairwise FST values between populations and by AMOVA, as implemented in the software ARLEQUIN v3.5. Significance levels were obtained with 10,000 permutations. Data were tested for the presence of isolation by distance (IBD) by regressing natural logarithm-transformed geographical distances between sampling sites (in km) against Slatkin's linearized FST (FST/(1-FST)). Statistical significance was assessed using a Mantel test with 10,000 permutations in ARLEQUIN. The six-bar mutational spectra (C•G→A•T, C•G→G•C, C•G→T•A, T•A→A•T, T•A→C•G and T•A→G•C) of haplotype were calculated using in-house script (available upon request). Each haplotype was compared with the sequence of earliest sample in 2014.

2.5. Phylogeographic analysis using RASP software

Phylogenetic tree of the haplotype was estimated using RAxML v8 with the GTR + gamma evolutionary model and 500 bootstrap replicates. The ML tree from RAxML analysis was then used as a starting tree for BEAST 1.8.1. The earliest time of individuals of each haplotype was used as tip date for dating. The analysis was done using the Yule Process for the tree prior and the uncorrelated lognormal (UCLD) relaxed clock model. We performed 200 million generations, sampling every 10,000 and generating 20,000 trees. The condensed tree was generated using TreeAnnotator v1.8.1 with a burn-in of 4000 trees. For the phylogeographic analyses, we used the S-DIVA (Statistical dispersal-vicariance analysis) method implemented in RASP software to analyse the ancestral geographic ranges of EBOV lineages. In S-DIVA analysis, 1000 random trees were generated from trees data set discarded the first 4000 trees. One hundred and 10,000 alternative reconstructions were kept for random trees and final tree, respectively. The alternative reconstruction with the maximal S-DIVA value was used for further analysis. The total number of dispersal and vicariance, dispersal curve and the dispersal among and within each district were calculated based on the best reconstruction in RASP.

3. Key findings regarding genetics of the 2013-2015 EBOV outbreak

Hap8 in multiple viral haplotypes is the major epidemic lineage in the 2014 Sierra Leone outbreak. This observation highlights how Ebola virus is substantially different in virulence or transmissibility in comparison to the virus lineages associated with 2014 outbreaks in Sierra Leone, which provides a clue to understand the 2014 EBOV spreading.

We first performed viral whole genomes of EBOV alignment using 305 available genomic data from 1976 to 2014, and then we did pairwise comparison of the gene coding regions (NP, VP35, VP40, GP, VP30, VP24, L) in the 305 viral genomes, which were used for phylogenetic tree analysis by MrBayes [9]. The condensed Bayesian tree reconstructed from this data matrix showed strongly supported relationships consistent with the results from previous reports [5]. In the **Figure S1A**, the phylogenetic comparison to all 19 genomes (Yellow) during earlier outbreaks before 2014 suggests that the EBOV during 2014 EVD epidemic likely spread from the central Africa within the past decade. These EBOV from Sierra Leone during September to November 2014 (Red) follow the same patterns as observed in individual EBOV sequences during the early outbreak from March to August 2014 (Blue), which are derived from 2014 Sierra Leone 2 and 2014 Sierra Leone 3 as described in early publication [3–5]. The distribution map represented the geographical distribution of the 175 newly sequenced individual samples of EBOV during September to November 2014 with different colours at five districts (47 samples in Western Urban, 67 in Western Rural, 47 in Port Loko, 5 in Kambia, and 9 in Bombali) (**Figure S1B**), which were further used in the phylogeographic analysis. Phylogenetic tree constructed using the maximum likelihood method [10] showed a similar topology with Bayesian tree [9] (**Figures S2** and **S3**). Since the evolution and the variations among genotypes of EBOV was suggested with an observed low rate in early publications [3, 4], we investigated the genomic portrait of haplotype diversity in EBOV from 1976 to 2014 [11]. In total, 176 different viral haplotypes were identified from the 305 viral coding sequences (**Figure 1A** and **Table S1**). The haplotype frequency distribution was strongly skewed, with the vast majority of haplotypes found only once (139 out of 176) and restricted to a single viral genome. Hap144,

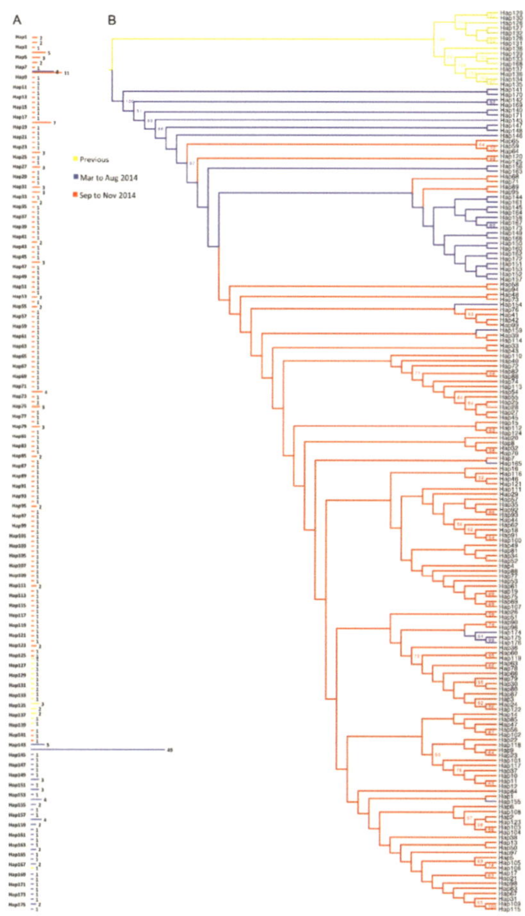

Figure 1. Multiple viral haplotypes of EBOV coexisted during the 2014 EVD outbreak. (A) The number of viral genomes in multiple viral haplotypes of EBOV (Histogram); (B) A maximum likelihood tree created with RAxML puts the 176 multiple viral haplotypes. The green values on the branch are the bootstrap values for corresponding nodes, only bootstrap values greater than 50 were shown.

which is the most common haplotype, includes 49 individuals from June 2014. The Hap8 including 19 viral sequences is the second common haplotype, which contains 8 individuals in the early outbreaks of 2014 and 11 individuals in the late outbreaks of 2014, respectively. A maximum likelihood tree of 176 haplotypes were represented in **Figure 1B**. Bootstrap values higher than 50% are shown for each node. The un-rooted ML tree revealed that there were no distinct haplotype groups with high bootstrap support.

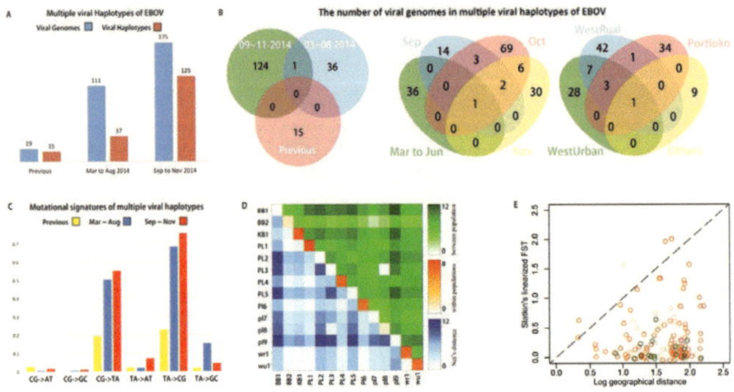

Figure 2. The mutational signatures and phylogeography analysis in multiple haplotypes of EBOV. (A) The 176 different viral haplotypes were identified in the 305 analysed genomes of EBOV; (B) The multiple viral haplotypes of EBOV with the temporal and spatial distribution (Venn); (C) The mutational signatures of multiple viral haplotypes; (D) Nei's distance (lower triangle) and Average pairwise distance (upper triangle) within and between the populations (BB, Bombali; KB, Kambia; PL, Port Loko; WR, Western Rural; WU, Western Urban.); (E) Isolation by distance plots of pairwise population values for log geographic distance (km) and genetic distance. Genetic distance is given by Slatkin's linearized FST (FST /(1- FST) Geographic distance is given in km.

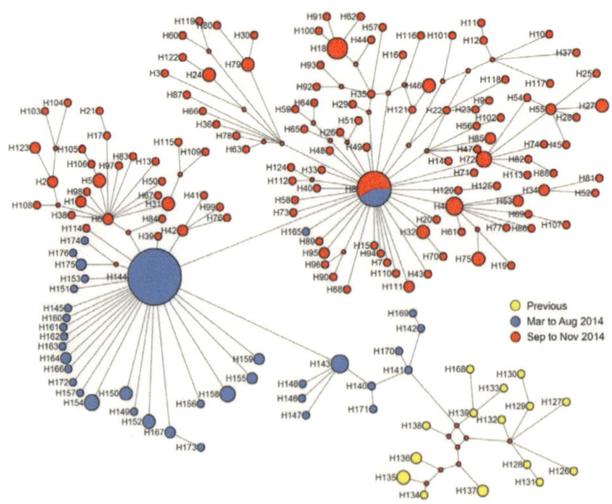

Figure 3. Median-joining haplotype network of multiple viral haplotypes in EBOV. The median-joining haplotype network covered the 176 multiple viral haplotypes of EBOV from 1976 to 2014; each circle represents a unique haplotype, and its size is proportional to its frequency.

In the **Figure 2A**, we found 15 different viral haplotypes in the 19 viral coding sequences in the previous outbreaks before 2014. In the 111 viral coding sequences during the earlier outbreak of 2014 (March to August, 2014), 37 different viral haplotypes were detected. Particularly, 125 different viral haplotypes were identified from the 175 viral coding sequences during September to November 2014. Interestingly, the Hap8 is the only one viral haplotype with the viral sequences that covers both early and late 2014 outbreaks in Sierra Leone (**Figure 2B**, the left Venn picture), which means that the Hap8 differentiated from the progenitor virus from June 2014 and maintained renewal to keep the population. Within the 11 individuals of Hap 8 from September to November 2014 (**Figure 2B**, the middle Venn picture), we found that 3 viral genomes from Western Urban, 2 viral genomes from Port Loko, 5 viral genomes from Bombali and one viral genome from Western Rural (**Figure 2B**, the right Venn picture), while all individuals of Hap144 are only represented in early outbreaks of 2014. This result implies that the Hap8 may be the major viral haplotype during 2014 Sierra Leone EVD epidemic.

3.1. Mutation types: EBOV mutations are typically C•G→T•A and T•A→C•G

The analyses of nucleotide substitutions as six-bar mutational spectra (C•G→A•T, C•G→G•C, C•G→T•A, T•A→A•T, T•A→C•G and T•A→G•C) have been proven useful in showing how mutational spectra can be specific to viral type and related to viral coding sequences. The analysis based on viral haplotypes has shown significant mutational signatures among their sequences (**Figure 2C**, **Figure S4** and **Table S2**). The results in **Figure 2C** indicated that the mutations of Ebola viruses are mainly C•G→T•A and T•A→C•G, and the nucleotide mutation rate during 2014 outbreak was much higher than the rate in previous.

3.2. Genetic characteristics are not correlated with geographical distance

We are interested in the relationship between the genetic distance in viral multiple haplotypes and the geographic distance (**Figure S1B**). In **Figure 2D**, we compared Nei's distance [12] (lower triangle) and Average pairwise distance [13] (upper triangle) within and between the populations (**Table S3**) during September to November 2014. The dark parts of lower triangle were mainly represented from PL2 to PL9, which suggested that the populations in Port Loko have higher genetic divergence than others. Population KB1, PL1, PL4, PL6, WR1 and WU1 represented high genetic distance within each of them, which suggested that these populations have higher genetic divergence within them. The isolation by distance (IBD) analyses [14] detected no positive correlation between genetic distance (Slatkin's linearized FST) and log geographical distance (**Figure 2E**) [15], and the p value of analyses mantel test is 0.459. This finding was consistent when we restrained the analysis within Port Loko, which included most populations. We also compared the pairwise distances from the sequences of 126 different viral haplotypes from September to November 2014 (**Figure S5**). Most of the haplotypes represent a low pairwise distances (less than 15) except Hap109 and Hap115. Both of the two haplotypes were represented in the tip of the haplotypes tree in **Figure 1B**, which indicated that they divided recently. The date of sampling for the two haplotypes was November 9th 2014, which support their position in evolutionary dynamic [3].

3.3. The evolution and variation between EBOV genotypes was low, which suggest that the viral haplotypes may be common in this transmission

In order to infer the connections of multiple viral haplotypes, we reconstructed a median joining haplotype network [16], which covered the 176 multiple viral haplotypes of EBOV (**Figure 3** and **Table S4**). The star-like network was characterized by a few common viral haplotypes, surrounded by many viral haplotypes mostly present in only 1–5 individuals (except Hap18). Most viral haplotype were divided between two haplotypes at opposite ends of the network. Thorough spatial mixing was evident, with the central haplotype (Hap8) being shared by 19 different viral coding sequences from March to November 2014 representing the major haplotype during the outbreak 2014.

In the **Figure 4A**, the haplotype network showed the main haplotypes, which contain more than 3 individuals in each. The relationship between the haplotype network and four sub-clades in 2014 outbreaks was identified in the phylogenetic tree, which was reconstructed

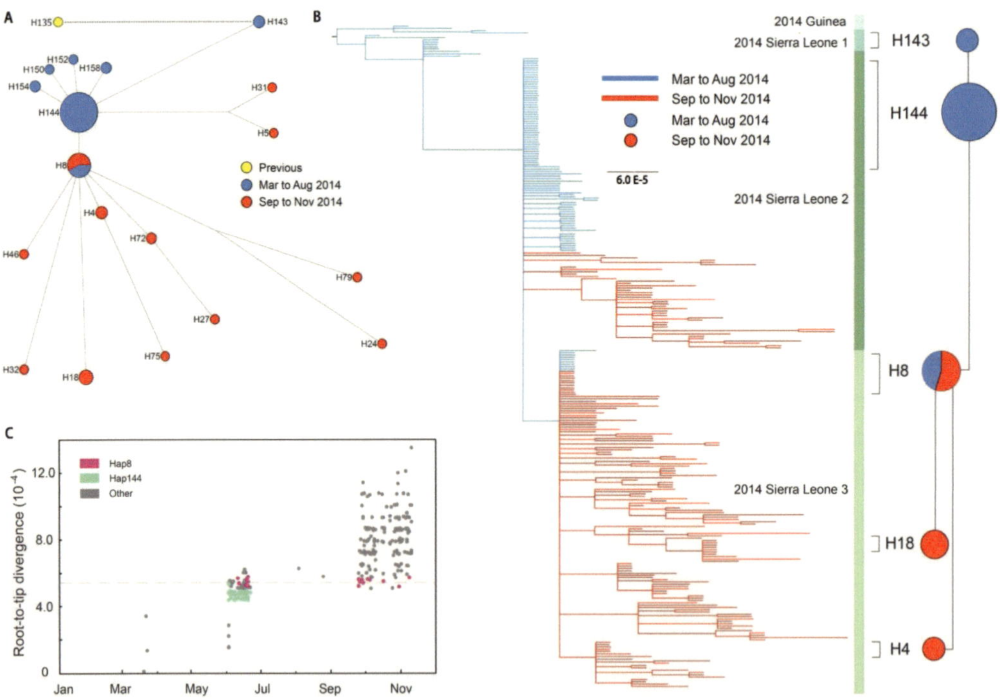

Figure 4. Main viral haplotypes in median joining haplotype network and phylogenetic analysis with outbreak in 2014. (A) Main haplotypes and those containing more than three viral genomes. Lines represent base pair changes between two haplotypes, with the length proportional to the number of base pair changes. Haplotypes and those containing island samples are labelled by name. (B) A Bayesian phylogenetic tree of EBOV lineages created by MrBayes with the main outbreak of viral haplotypes in 2014 on the left. (C) Root-to-tip divergence of each sample plotting with corresponding collection date. The estimates were based on ML tree and the root was placed on the common ancestral branch of Guinea strains. Strains of Hap 8, Hap 144 and other haplotypes were coloured magenta, cyan and grey.

by 286 viral sequences in 2014 outbreak (**Figure 4B**). The viral genomes during September to November 2014 mainly belong to Sierra Leone 3, despite some located in the Sierra Leone 2. The circles and lines alongside the tree tips indicate the corresponding common haplotypes and their relationships in the median joining haplotype network. Importantly, combining this network, we found that the 49 individuals of Hap144 from June 2014 were only located in the sub-lineage, Sierra Leone 2, while all 19 individuals of Hap8 from June to November 2014 were located in the sub-clade Sierra Leone 3. We did root-to-tip analysis by Maximum Likelihood tree rooted on the common ancestor of Guinea branches. The result of root-to-tip distances suggests that the viral genomes during September to November 2014 displayed high divergence and there appeared to be an increase in the viral diversity in **Figure 4C**. Despite the high-diversified viral sequences, the Hap8 still kept its stable rate and circulated nearly half the year. Thus, the Hap8 maintained a stable state from June to November 2014, which supported our hypothesis that the Hap8 is the major lineage in 2014 Sierra Leone EVD outbreak.

3.4. Analyses showed that the Western rural region was the dispersal and differentiation centre for EBOV in Sierra Leone

Based on the phylogenetic relationship of viral haplotypes, we analysed the phylogeographic distribution [17, 18] of the EBOV during September to November 2014 in Sierra Leone with their detailed geographic information. The viral haplotypes tree with optimal reconstruction of highest S-DIVA Value is shown in **Figure 4A** [19, 20]. Pie charts reflect probability of the respective area and areas are colour-coded as well as the legends allowing for single or combined distributions. The reconstruction reveals at least 63 dispersals and 46 variances to explain the present distribution pattern of the EBOV. The results indicated that the ancestor of the outbreak from September to November 2014 had originated in the Western Rural and Western Urban (75% support, node 249). The tree then divided into two major clades, one originated in Western Rural (node 248) and the other originated in Western Urban (node 153). The red highlight clade in **Figure 5A** represented the dispersal routes of Hap 8, which starts from Western Rural, and then disperses to Port Loko and other districts. The dispersal routes of all samples in Hap 8 are represented in **Figure S6**, which support dispersal routes of Hap 8. The diagram of dispersal events (blue line) and node density (green line) is represented in **Figure 5B**. The total number of immigration, emigration and the divergence of haplotype of each province were represented in **Figure 5C**, which revealed that the emigration and divergence in Western Rural were much higher than other place, suggesting that Western Rural is likely to have been the source of the EBOV, which was in accordance with the epidemiological findings. The circle in **Figure 5D** showed the number of dispersals among Bombali, Kambia, Port Loko, Western Rural and Western Urban. It is interesting that The EBOV in Kambia came from Western Urban and Western Rural directly and there is no migration between Kambia and Port Loko or Kambia and Bombali. The green points in geographical map (**Figure 5D**) represented the distribution of Hap 8, which had a wide distribution in Bombali, Port Loko, Western Urban and Western Rual.

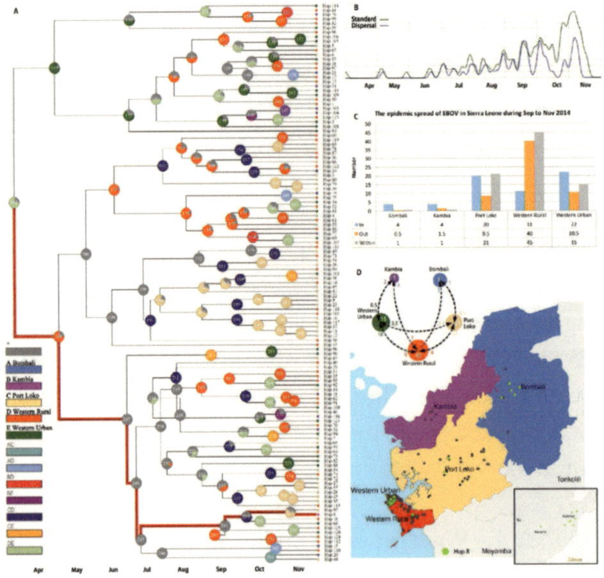

Figure 5. Phylogeographic analysis of the epidemic spread of Ebola virus in Sierra Leone. (A) Results of the biogeographic analysis of haplotypes using S-DIVA method. Pie charts show the probability values of the ancestral areas reconstructed at each node. Areas are colour-coded as in the legends allowing for single or combined distributions. (B) The diagram of dispersal events (blue line) and node density (green line) (C) The total number of immigration (in), emigration (out) and the divergence (within) of haplotype of each districts (D) The circle represented the number of dispersals among Bombali, Kambia, Port Loko, Western Rural and Western Urban. Map to show the geographical distribution of the districts of EBOV from September to November 2014. The distribution of Hap8 was highlighted with green points. We obtained the boundary data of the District from the GADM database of Global Administrative Areas version 2.0 (http://www.gadm.org), and the map was created in ArcGIS 9.2 software (ESRI Inc., Redlands, CA, USA).

4. Conclusions

Previously characterized EBOV strains were found to be substantially different in terms of virulence and transmissibility compared to the 2014 Sierra Leona lineage.

The EBOV epidemic from 2013 is having a devastating impact in West Africa. Collectively, in the previous study, they found the mutation sites of the sequenced EBOV genomes during March to November 2014 [1, 3–5], which generated genetically distinct sub-clades in Sierra Leone outbreak, following the emergence of multiple novel lineages of EBOV. Based on them, the sequencing genomes of EBOV has revealed extensive genetic variation [3,21], leading to speculation that the viral genomes have multiple viral haplotype in EBOV with the signatures of phylogeographic distribution during the 2014 EVD epidemic in Sierra Leone. It is implied that a genetically diverse multiple viral haplotypes of EBOV governs the 2014 EVD epidemic.

The lack of functional distinction between the previous and 2014 Ebola outbreaks emphasizes the importance of the diversity multiple viral haplotypes [5, 22]. Here we analysed the multiple viral haplotypes in the coding sequences of EBOV from 1976 to 2014 outbreaks. In the 176

multiple viral haplotypes during the 2014 outbreak (**Figure 1**), although the Hap144 is the most common haplotype, the Hap8 is the major viral haplotype with the long temporal and extensive spatial distribution during 2014 EVD outbreaks in Sierra Leone (**Figure 2** and **4**). The reconstructed median join network of multiple viral haplotypes displayed a "star-like" shape with no deep branching among haplotypes (**Figure 3**), which shows the similarity topology in the each outbreak with the most common haplotypes in the centre. It demonstrates the high degree of similarity of the progenitor virus of each outbreak, which suggests that future transmissions of similarly virulent potential are highly likely [3, 5, 23].

We also found evidence that the multiple viral haplotypes in EBOV have the significant mutational signatures (**Figure 2C** and **S4**). Interestingly, the mutations associated with smoking-related damage in lung cancers are mainly C•G→A•T transversions [24], whereas mutations associated with ultraviolet (UV) radiation exposure in skin cancers comprise predominantly C•G→T•A transitions [25]. Strategies for containing EBOV in West Africa have been suggested, but are predicated on lack of adaptation of the virus. These results indicate that the mutational signatures in multiple viral haplotypes of EBOV may be cause by the chemomorphosis and the environment of ultraviolet (UV) radiation.

Viral epidemics can develop strong growth heterogeneity even though the temporal and spatial scales of its initial outbreak are short.

In the 2014 Ebola epidemic, we have identified a genetic variant that has a substantially higher growth rate than its progenitor lineage [4, 21, 26]. We conclude that a viral epidemic can develop strong growth heterogeneity even on the limited temporal and spatial scales of its initial outbreak. If that heterogeneity has a genetic cause, our analysis suggests that selection can shape a fast-evolving pathogen on the time scales of a single epidemic. However, the viral genomes in the Hap8 had a stable growth rate. If this growth heterogeneity remains stable, it will generate major shifts in multiple viral haplotypes frequencies and influence the overall epidemic dynamics on time scales within the current outbreak. Thus, the long temporal distribution and stable evolution of the Hap8 indicated that it replaced Hap144 and further became the major epidemic haplotype in the year.

The difference between the 2014 outbreak and those that have occurred previously is the establishment of infections in relatively densely populated areas compared with previous outbreaks [27]. The genetic flow in EBOV was no more likely to occur between populations than among populations (**Figure 2D**). Overall, IBD analyses showed that there are no detected positive correlation between genetic and log geographical distance (**Figure 2E**). Our findings suggest that population growth, urbanization and immigration along the main road in Sierra Leone have created efficient pathways for EBOV transmission. The phylogeographic analyses showed the ancestor distribution of the outbreak from March to November 2014. Western Rural is the dispersal centre and differentiation centre of the Ebola virus, which not only spread virus to all other districts, but also generated the most haplotype (**Figure 4C**). In **Figure 4B**, the peaks of dispersal curve are (blue) below the node curve (red) most of the time except in the beginning of July and the middle of September 2014. This result indicated that there may have been small-scale outbreaks during these periods.

Further analysis of these differences may help to explain how the 2013-2015 outbreak spread so rapidly and widely. Genetic data will be able to yield insights into the evolutionary dynamics of EBOV.

In summary, our study first detected the diversity of multiple viral haplotypes in EBOV with systematic calculation of phylogeographic distribution. We found that the haplotype, Hap8, is the major epidemic lineage in the 2014 Sierra Leone outbreak. The mutations of Ebola viruses are mainly C•G→T•A and T•A→C•G, and the nucleotide mutation rate during 2014 outbreak was much higher than the rate in previous outbreaks. Moreover, the continuously increasing genetic diversity of the 2014 EBOV were also found in our result. The genetic flow in EBOV was no more likely to occur within or without populations and the correlation between genetic and log geographical distance is not significant. However, Western Rural is the dispersal centre and differentiation centre of the Ebola virus in Sierra Leone. Our method is based on simple summary statistics of multiple viral haplotypes, which can be inferred from genealogical trees with an underlying lineage-specific model of the infection dynamics. However, all analysis of haplotype diversity and phylogeographic distribution starting from the initial phase of an epidemic are probabilistic extrapolations; they are based on limited data and subject to confounding factors such as variation in sampling density [28]. As more sequence data emerge, updated haplotype diversity and phylogeographic distribution will suggest targets for detailed epidemiological investigation and provide predictive insight into the dynamics of the epidemic.

5. Limitations

Analyses of haplotype diversity and phylogeographic distribution are probabilistic extrapolations based on limited data as a result of the intrinsic difficulty in collecting samples.

A range of confounding factors is also implicit, such as variations in sampling density.

Acknowledgements

This work was supported by a grant from the State Key Laboratory of Pathogen and BioSecurity Program (No. SKLPBS1408 and No. SKLPBS1451).

Authors' contributions

Y.T., Y.Y., and Y.J. characterized the materials, under the supervision of Y.T., Y.Y., and D.F. wrote the manuscript with further contributions from J.Y. and X.P.A. analysed the data. All authors reviewed the manuscript.

Additional information

Competing financial interests and the authors declare no competing financial interests.

Author details

Yue Teng[1*], Yan Yu[2,3], Yuan Jin[1], Xiaoping An[1] and Dan Feng[4*]

*Address all correspondence to: yueteng@me.com and fddd@263.net

1 State Key Laboratory of Pathogen and Biosecurity, Beijing, China

2 Key Laboratory of Bio-Resources and Eco-Environment of Ministry of Education, College of Life Sciences, Sichuan University, Sichuan Province, China

3 Department of Biology, Duke University, Durham, USA

4 Division of Standard Operational Management, Institute of Hospital Management, Chinese PLA General Hospital, Beijing, China

Yue Teng, Yan Yu and Yuan Jin contributed equally to this work.

References

[1] Baize S., *et al*. Emergence of Zaire Ebola Virus Disease in Guinea. *N Engl J Med*. 371, 1418–1425 (2014)

[2] World Health Organization. One year into the Ebola epidemic: a deadly, tenacious and unforgiving virus. http://www.who.int/csr/disease/ebola/one-year-report/introduction/en/

[3] Tong Y.G., *et al*. Genetic Diversity and Evolutionary Dynamics of Ebola Virus in Sierra Leone. *Nature*. (Accepted, doi:10.1038/nature14490, 2015)

[4] Hoenen T., et al. Mutation rate and genotype variation of Ebola virus from Mali case sequences. *Science*. 348, 117–119 (2015)

[5] Gire S.K., *et al*. Genomic surveillance elucidates Ebola virus origin and transmission during the 2014 outbreak. *Science*. 345, 1369–1372 (2014)

[6] Agnandji S.T., et al. Phase 1 Trials of rVSV Ebola Vaccine in Africa and Europe – Preliminary Report. *N Engl J Med*. 2015 Apr 1. [Epub ahead of print]. DOI: 10.1056/NEJMoa1414216

[7] Regules J. A., et al. A Recombinant Vesicular Stomatitis Virus Ebola Vaccine - Preliminary Report. *N Engl J Med*. 2015 Apr 1. [Epub ahead of print]. DOI: 10.1056/NEJMoa1414216

[8] Marzi A., et al. An Ebola whole-virus vaccine is protective in nonhuman primates. *Science*. 2015 Mar 26. [Epub ahead of print]. DOI: 10.1126/science.aaa4919

[9] Ronquist F., Huelsenbeck J. P. MrBayes 3: Bayesian phylogenetic inference under mixed models. *Bioinformatics*. 19, 1572–1574 (2003)

[10] Stamatakis A. RAxML version 8: a tool for phylogenetic analysis and post-analysis of large phylogenies. *Bioinformatics*. 30, 1312–1313 (2014)

[11] Kortenhoeven C. Virus genome dynamics under different propagation pressures: reconstruction of whole genome haplotypes of west Nile viruses from NGS data. *BMC Genomics*. 16, 118 (2015)

[12] Nei M. Molecular Evolutionary Genetics. Columbia University Press, New York, NY, USA. (1987)

[13] Tajima F. Evolutionary relationship of DNA sequences in finite populations. *Genetics*. 105, 437–460 (1983)

[14] Peel A. J., *et al*. Continent-wide panmixia of an African fruit bat facilitates transmission of potentially zoonotic viruses. *Nature communications*. 4, 2770 (2013)

[15] Slatkin M. A measure of population subdivision based on microsatellite allele frequencies. *Genetics*. 139,457–462 (1995)

[16] Bandelt H. J., Forster P., Röhl A. Median-joining networks for inferring intraspecific phylogenies. *Mol Biol Evol*. 16, 37–48 (1999)

[17] Excoffier L., Lischer H. E. L. Arlequin suite ver 3.5: a new series of programs to perform population genetics analyses under Linux and Windows. *Mol Ecol Resour*. 10, 564–567 (2010).

[18] Rozas J., et al. DnaSP, DNA polymorphism analyses by the coalescent and other methods. *Bioinformatics*. 19, 2496–2497 (2003)

[19] Yu Y., et al. RASP (Reconstruct Ancestral State in Phylogenies): a tool for historical biogeography. *Mol Phylogenet Evol*. 87, 46–49 (2015)

[20] Yu Y., Harris A. J., He X. S-DIVA (Statistical Dispersal-Vicariance Analysis): A tool for inferring biogeographic histories. *Mol Phylogenet Evol*. 56, 848–850 (2010)

[21] Vogel G. Infectious Diseases. A reassuring snapshot of Ebola. *Science*. 347, 1407 (2015)

[22] Scarpino S. V. Epidemiological and viral genomic sequence analysis of the 2014 Ebola outbreak reveals clustered transmission. *Clin Infect Dis*. 60, 1079–1082 (2015)

[23] Dowall S. D., et al. Elucidating variations in the nucleotide sequence of Ebola virus associated with increasing pathogenicity. *Genome Biol*. 15, 540 (2014)

[24] Helleday T. Mechanisms underlying mutational signatures in human cancers. *Nat Rev Genet*. 15, 585–598 (2014)

[25] Pfeifer G. P., You Y. H., Besaratinia A. Mutations induced by ultraviolet light. *Mutat Res*. 571, 19–31 (2005).

[26] Alizon S. Quantifying the epidemic spread of Ebola virus (EBOV) in Sierra Leone using phylodynamics. *Virulence*. 5, 825–827 (2014)

[27] Goeijenbier M. Ebola virus disease: a review on epidemiology, symptoms, treatment and pathogenesis. *Neth J Med*. 72, 442–448 (2014)

[28] Kugelman J. R. Evaluation of the potential impact of Ebola virus genomic drift on the efficacy of sequence-based candidate therapeutics. *MBio*. 6 (2015)

Chapter 5

Prediction of Ebolavirus Genomes Encoded MicroRNA-Like Small RNAs Using Bioinformatics Approaches

Yue Teng, Zhe Xu, Jin Yuan, Xiaoping An,
Jiangman Song and Dan Feng

Additional information is available at the end of the chapter

http://dx.doi.org/10.5772/62944

Abstract

Recent findings revealed that certain viruses encoded microRNA-like small RNAs using the RNA interference machinery in the host cells. However, the function of these virus-encoded microRNA-like small RNAs remained unclear, and whether these microRNA-like small RNAs were involved in the replication of the virus and viral infection was still disputable. In this chapter, the negative-sense RNA genome of Ebola virus (EBOV) was scanned using bioinformatics tools to predict the EBOV-encoded microRNA-like small RNAs. Then, the potential influence of viral microRNA-like small RNAs on the viral immune evasion, host cellular signaling pathway, and epigenetic regulation of antiviral defense mechanism were also detected by the reconstructed regulatory network of target genes associated with viral encoded microRNA-like small RNAs. In this analysis, EBOV-encoded microRNA-like small RNAs were proposed to inhibit the host immune response factors, probably facilitating the evasion of EBOV from the host defense mechanisms. In conclusion, systematic investigation of microRNA-like small RNAs in EBOV genome may shed light on the underlying molecular mechanisms of the pathological process of Ebola virus disease (EVD).

Keywords: Ebolavirus, virus-encoded miRNAs, microRNAs, bioinformatics, NF-kB, TNF

1. Introduction

Zaire Ebola virus (ZEBOV) has the highest case-fatality rate with an average of approximately 83% over the past 27 years [1]. Its first outbreak took place on August 26, 1976, in Yambuku [2], and the virus was also responsible for the 2014 West Africa outbreak, which was the largest

EBOV outbreak in record [3–6]. Moreover, neither antiviral drugs nor effective treatment was available for EBOV or Ebola virus disease (EVD) at that time [7, 8]. MicroRNAs originate from a wide variety of primary transcripts (pri-miRNAs) that are generated by RNA polymerase II (pol II) in all eukaryotes [9] or by RNA polymerase III (pol III) in some viruses [10]. The cleavage of pri-miRNAs releases a RNA hairpin intermediate (~70 nt) containing a characteristic 2 nt 3′ overhang, named a premature miRNA (pre-miRNA), which is further processed to generate the 21~23 nt mature miRNA from its arm of ~70 nt imperfect stem-loop structure [11, 12].

Since microRNAs have been discovered and their role in gene expression regulation was established, it has been hypothesized that viruses could encode microRNA-like small RNAs as well, and these virus-encoded microRNA-like small RNAs were proposed to play important regulatory roles in viral immune evasion and systemic pathogenesis [13–15]. The size of viral encoded microRNA-like RNAs has a significant advantage given the tight constraints on viral genome size, which is also small enough to escape from the triggered host immune pathway. It was found that viral encoded microRNA-like small RNAs could downregulate the expression of host immune defense gene, resulting in increased viral replication or evasion from host immune surveillance [16, 17]. Until now, more than 60 viral microRNA-like small RNAs have been identified [18–24], most of which came from Herpes virues [25]. Only a small part of such RNAs was detected within Retrovirus, Adenovirus, and polyomavirus families [26–28].

Bioinformatics-driven prediction was an effective method to identify viral encoded microRNA-like small RNAs [21, 22]. In this study, the microRNA prediction program, VMir, was applied to scan the viral genomes for the presence of stem-loop structures in the pri- and pre-miRNAs and identify potential candidate stretches capable to form stable secondary stem-loop structures. Afterward, putative mature microRNA-like small RNAs were validated using MatureBayes [29]. The systemic prediction of the potential EBOV-encoded microRNA-like small RNAs along with their target genes on the genome-wide scale helps to further assess the function of microRNAs during viral infection and virus-host interactions in the EVD pathogenesis.

2. Methods

2.1. EBOV whole genome sequences and alignment

The full-length genome sequences of EBOV were retrieved from the genome browser at Ebola virus resource (http://www.ncbi.nlm.nih.gov/genome/viruses/variation/ebola/) and UCSC Ebola portal (https://genome.ucsc.edu/ebolaPortal/). MAFFT Multiple Sequence Alignment Software Version 7 were applied for the alignment of the EBOV genomes [30].

2.2. Bioinformatics prediction of the EBOV genome-encoded microRNA-like small RNAs

Briefly, the viral genome was scanned for stem-loop structures of miRNA precursor (pre-miRNA) using VMir [31] with default parameter settings (http://www.hpi-hamburg.de/research/departments-and-research-groups/antiviral-defense-mechanism/software-down-

http://dx.doi.org/10.5772/62944

load.html). The putative pre-miRNAs with VMir score ≥150 and a window count ≥ 35 were retained. Then, MiPred software [32] was applied to check all of the putative miRNA precursors, and precursors with confidence equal to or greater than 70% were further analyzed. Subsequently, mature miRNA sequences were predicted from the putative pre-miRNA stem-loops. Finally, the MatureBayes tool [29] was used to extend the prediction coverage of the mature miRNAs under default parameter settings.

2.3. Prediction of the target genes and signaling pathway analysis

Target genes of predicted EBOV-encoded microRNA-like small RNAs in the human genome were predicted using TargetScan [33]. Putative targets within the viral genome were predicted using TargetScan Perl script. The signaling pathways collected from the Kyoto Encyclopedia of Genes and Genomes (KEGG) [34–36] PATHWAY databases were applied in the pathway analysis.

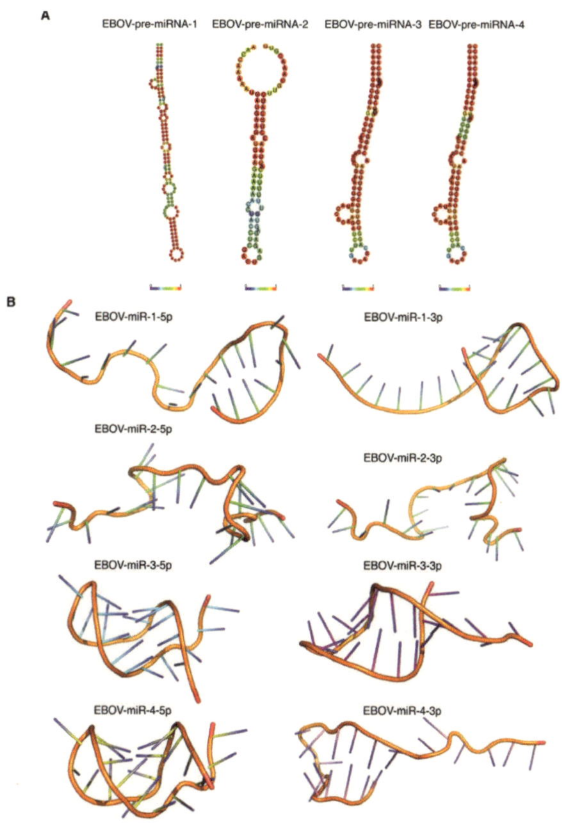

Figure 1. The predicted EBOV-encoded pre-miRNAs and microRNA-like small RNAs. The MiPred algorithm was used to identify genuine pre-miRNAs, and the MatureBayes tool was used to predict the mature miRNA sequences. (A) The secondary structures of the four EBOV pre-miRNAs. (B) The tertiary structures of the EBOV-encoded micro-RNA-like small RNAs.

2.4. Constructing gene regulation network

The genetic regulation network was constructed based on systematic integration of various datasets. Transcription factors related with the target genes of EBOV-encoded microRNA-like small RNAs were selected from Transcriptional Regulatory Element Database (TRED) [37–39]. The integrated regulatory network of target genes with transcription factors was constructed using Cytoscape software (http://cytoscape.org/).

3. Key findings regarding the bioinformatics prediction of EBOV genome-encoded microRNA-like small RNAs

3.1. Predicted precursor and mature EBOV genome-encoded microRNA-like small RNAs

The released full-length genome sequences of the retrieved EBOV strains were aligned and then scanned for miRNA precursor (pre-miRNA) using VMir software. Afterward, the putative pre-miRNAs with VMir score ≥150 and a window count ≥35 were selected for further assessment. Within the EBOV genome, four putative microRNA precursors, EBOV-pre-miRNA-1, EBOV-pre-miRNA-2, EBOV-pre-miRNA-3, and EBOV-pre-miRNA-4 were predicted (**Figure 1A**). The mature miRNA sequences were predicted from the putative pre-miRNA stem loops. Seven different mature EBOV miRNA candidates, including EBOV-miR-1-5p, EBOV-miR-1-3p, EBOV-miR-2-5p, EBOV-miR-2-3p, EBOV-miR-3-5p, EBOV-miR-3-3p, EBOV-miR-4-5p, and EBOV-miR-4-3p were resolved using MatureBayes tool (**Figure 1B**).

3.2. Bioinformatics analysis of the genetic regulation network in the target genes of EBOV genome-encoded microRNA-like small RNAs

Target genes of the predicted mature microRNA-like small RNAs were searched within TargetScan, and the potential target genes in host were identified (**Table S1**, the list of potential target genes of EBOV-encoded microRNA-like small RNAs). KEGG pathway enrichment analysis was performed using the DAVID bioinformatics tool for these target genes. The results showed that the target genes were closely related on function and were involved in multiple canonical pathways, such as NF-kB activation by viruses, role of protein kinase (PKR) in interferon induction and antiviral response, induction of apoptosis by HIV1, B cell-activating factor signaling, and role of PI3K/AKT signaling in the pathogenesis of influenza, which were important in human immune response to virus infection (**Table 1**).

Canonical pathways	p-Value	Ratio	Molecules
AMPK signaling	*1.49E+00*	*2.26E-02*	*PDRK1, FASN, ADRA2B, RRKAB2*
Angiopoietin signaling	*4.47E-01*	*1.54E-02*	*NFKBIE*
April mediated signaling	*6.43E-01*	*2.63E-02*	*NFKBIE*
ATM signaling	*4.81E-01*	*1.69E-02*	*MRE11A*

Canonical pathways	p-Value	Ratio	Molecules
B cell activating factor signaling	*6.24E-01*	*2.5E-02*	*NFKBIE*
B cell receptor signaling	*4.92E-01*	*1.17E-02*	*PDPK1, NFKBIE*
CD27 signaling in lymphocytes	*5.34E-01*	*1.96E-02*	*NFKBIE*
CD28 signaling in t helper cells	*7.5E-01*	*1.77E-02*	*PDPK1, NFKBIE*
CD40 signaling	*4.53E-01*	*1.56E-02*	*NFKBIE*
bf2 signaling	*4.89E-01*	*1.16E-02*	*PDPK1, EIF2AK4*
ErbB signaling	*3.58E-01*	*1.18E-02*	*PDPK1*
ErbB2-ErbB3 signaling	*5E-01*	*1.79E-02*	*PDPK1*
ErbB4 signaling	*4.87E-01*	*1.72E-02*	*PDPK1*
Erythropoietin signaling	*1.12E+00*	*2.99E-02*	*PDPK1, NFKBIE*
HGF signaling	*2.95E-01*	*9.62E-03*	*ELF3*
HIF1a signaling	*3.07E-01*	*1E-02*	*MMP25*
IGF-1 signaling	*1.55E+00*	*3.09E-02*	*GRB10, PDPK1, SOCS4*
IL-1 signaling	*8.99E-01*	*2.2E-02*	*GNAT1, NFKBIE*
IL-10 signaling	*4.32E-01*	*1.47E-02*	*NFKBIE*
IL-17A signaling in airway cells	*4.53E-01*	*1.56E-02*	*NFKBIE*
IL-17A signaling in fibroblasts	*6.75E-01*	*2.86E-02*	*NFKBIE*
il-6 signaling	*2.63E-01*	*8.62E-03*	*NFKBIE*
Induction of apoptosis by HIV1	*1.22E+00*	*3.39E-02*	*NFKBIE, RIPK1*
Insulin receptor signaling	*6.69E-01*	*1.56E-02*	*GRB10, PDPK1*
JAK/Stat signaling	*4.12E-01*	*1.39E-02*	*SOCS4*
Lymphotoxin β receptor signaling	*5.13E-01*	*1.85E-02*	*PDPK1*
MIF regulation of innate immunity	*6.14E-01*	*2.44E-02*	*NFKBIE*
mTOR signaling	*4.57E-01*	*1.1E-02*	*PDPK1, PRKAB2*
NF-KB activation by viruses	*1.06E+00*	*2.74E-02*	*NFKBIE, RIPK1*
NF-KB signaling	*4.99E-01*	*1.18E-02*	*NFKBIE, RIPK1*
NGF signaling	*2.89E-01*	*9.43E-03*	*PDPK1*
P53 signaling	*3.13E-01*	*1.02E-02*	*CCND2*
PI3K signaling in B lymphocytes	*6.94E-01*	*1.63E-02*	*PDPK1, NFKBIE*
PI3K/AKT signaling	*7.05E-01*	*1.65E-02*	*PDPK1, NFKBIE*
PKCθ signaling in T lymphocytes	*2.71E-01*	*8.85E-03*	*NFKBIE*
PPARa/RXRa activation	*9.95E-01*	*1.82E-02*	*FASN, NFKBIE, PRKAB2*
Regulation of IL-2 expression in activated and anergic T lymphocytes	*3.86E-01*	*1.28E-02*	*NFKBIE*

Canonical pathways	p-Value	Ratio	Molecules
Role of IL-17A in arthritis	*5.13E-01*	*1.85E-02*	*NFKBIE*
Role of NFAT in regulation of the immune response	*5.1E-01*	*1.2E-02*	*GNAT1, NFKBIE*
Role of PI3K/AKT signaling in the pathogenesis of influenza	*4.75E-01*	*1.67E-02*	*NFKBIE*
Role of PKR in interferon induction and antiviral response	*6.24E-01*	*2.5E-02*	*NFKBIE*
STAT3 pathway	*4.08E-01*	*1.37E-02*	*SOCS4*
TNFR1 signaling	*1.4E+00*	*4.26E-02*	*NFKBIE, RIPK1*
TNFR2 signaling	*7.62E-01*	*3.57E-02*	*NFKBIE*
AMPK signaling	*1.49E+00*	*2.26E-02*	*PDPK1, FASN, ADRA2B, PRKAB2*
Angiopoietin signaling	*4.47E-01*	*1.54E-02*	*NFKBIE*
April mediated signaling	*6.43E-01*	*2.63E-02*	*NFKBIE*
ATM signaling	*4.81E-01*	*1.69E-02*	*MRE11A*
B cell activating factor signaling	*6.24E-01*	*2.5E-02*	*NFKBIE*
B cell receptor signaling	*4.92E-01*	*1.17E-02*	*PDPK1, NFKBIE*
CD27 signaling in lymphocytes	*5.34E-01*	*1.96E-02*	*NFKBIE*
CD28 signaling in T helper cells	*7.5E-01*	*1.77E-02*	*PDPK1, NFKBIE*
CD40 signaling	*4.53E-01*	*1.56E-02*	*NFKBIE*
EIF2 signaling	*4.89E-01*	*1.16E-02*	*PDPK1, EIF2AK4*
ErbB signaling	*3.58E-01*	*1.18E-02*	*PDPK1*
ErbB2-ErbB3 signaling	*5E-01*	*1.79E-02*	*PDPK1*
ErbB4 signaling	*4.87E-01*	*1.72E-02*	*PDPK1*
Erythropoietin signaling	*1.12E+00*	*2.99E-02*	*PDPK1, NFKBIE*
HGF signaling	*2.95E-01*	*9.62E-03*	*ELF3*
HIF1a signaling	*3.07E-01*	*1E-02*	*MMP25*
IGF-1 signaling	*1.55E+00*	*3.09E-02*	*GRB10, PDPK1, SOCS4*
IL-1 signaling	*8.99E-01*	*2.2E-02*	*GNAT1, NFKBIE*
IL-10 signaling	*4.32E-01*	*1.47E-02*	*NFKBIE*
IL-17A signaling in airway cells	*4.53E-01*	*1.56E-02*	*NFKBIE*
IL-17A signaling in fibroblasts	*6.75E-01*	*2.86E-02*	*NFKBIE*
IL-6 signaling	*2.63E-01*	*8.62E-03*	*NFKBIE*
Induction of apoptosis by HIV1	*1.22E+00*	*3.39E-02*	*NFKBIE, RIPK1*

Table 1. Key canonical pathway analysis of the potential mature EBOV miRNA target genes.

http://dx.doi.org/10.5772/62944

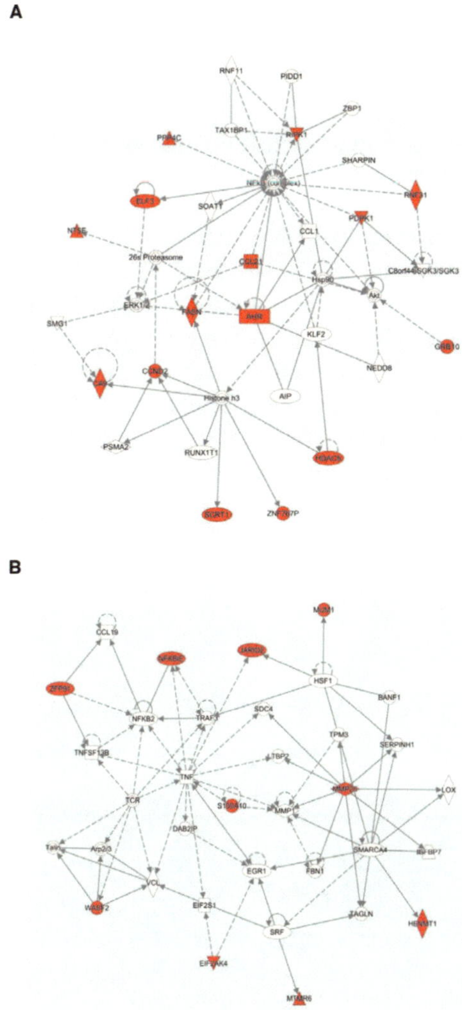

Figure 2. Bioinformatics analysis of the genetic regulatory network of target genes of EBOV-encoded microRNA-like small RNAs (A and B). The key regulation network of the potential target genes of EBOV-encoded microRNA-like small RNAs.

Based on the gene regulation network (GRN) analysis (Figure S1), it was found that target genes, FASN, RUNX1T1, and ELF3, were important immune and inflammation response factors and actively interacted with transcription regulator, such as KLF2 and NF-kB in host cells (**Figure 2A**) [40, 41]. They were also the key co-regulator of TNF complex in human immune system (**Figure 2B**) [42], implying that the EBOV might inhibit the infection response of immune system by affecting the related signaling pathway using noncoding RNA. Furthermore, it was speculated that the mature EBOV-encoded microRNA-like small RNAs might induce large-scale epigenetic modification in host genome to downregulate the expression of epigenetic factor, such as histone h3, HDAC5, JARID2, and SMARCA4, resulting in the inactivation of immune signaling and immune system with the antiviral response (**Figure 2A** and **2B**) [40–45].

3.3. Potential EBOV genome-encoded microRNA-like small RNAs associated with the Immune response-related pathways

Additionally, NF-kB and RIPK were also involved in the RIG-I-like receptor pathway (**Figure 3**) [46, 47]. As shown in **Figure 3**, the RIG-I-like receptor pathway played a key role in antiviral response that is a sensor for viruses such as influenza A, Rhabdovirus, Flavivirus, Paramyxovirus, Epstein-Barr virus, and Filovirus [48]. The RIG-I-like receptor pathway is stimulated during RNA virus infection by the interaction between cytosolic RIG-I and viral RNA structures that contain short hairpin dsRNA and 5′ triphosphate (5′ppp) terminal structure. The EBOV might utilize the microRNA-like small RNAs to inhibit the RIG-I-like receptor pathway to evade the host defense mechanisms, or conversely to trigger apoptosis responses as a

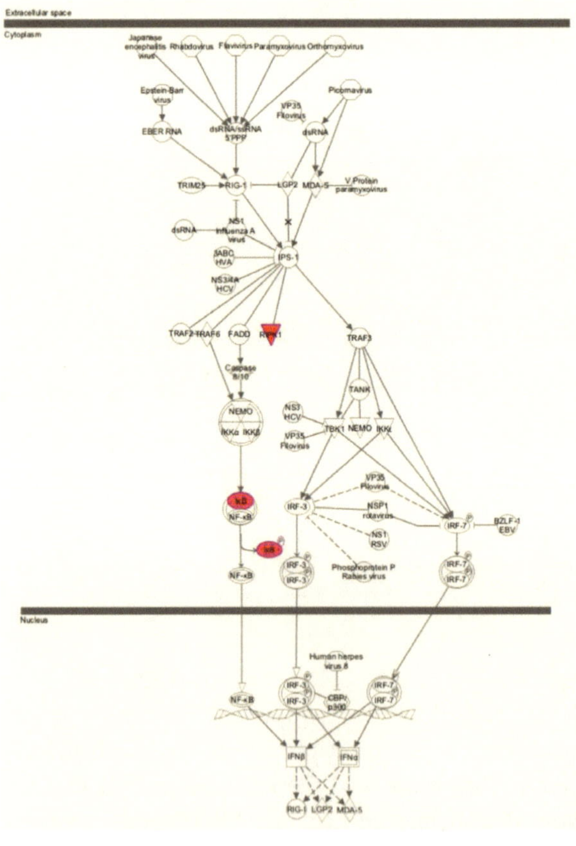

Figure 3. The RIG1I like receptor pathway associated with the potential target genes of EBOV-encoded microRNA1-like small RNAs. The target genes of EBOV-encoded microRNA1-like small RNAs, NF1kB, and RIPK, were involved in the RIG1I-like receptor pathway to trigger IFN signaling pathway with the antiviral response.

mechanism to increase viral infection [49, 50]. For viruses, effective RIG-I-mediated antiviral responses are dependent on functionally active LGP2. The dysfunction of LGP2 resulted in promoting viral replication, preventing virus-induced apoptosis, and suppressing the immune response for the invading pathogen [51]. Certain retroviruses, such as HIV-1, encode a protease that directs RIG-1 to the lysosome for degradation, and thereby evade RIG-1 mediated signaling. RIG-I and MDA-5 are involved in activating interferon (IFN) signaling pathway with the antiviral response.

4. Conclusions

MicroRNAs are encoded by cellular or viral genomes and play an essential role in numerous cellular processes, including viral infection, viral immune evasion, and antiviral cell-mediated immune response. Most viral genome-encoded microRNA-like small RNAs have been identified by traditional cloning strategy from virus-infected cells, yet others have been identified following computational prediction. Using the VMir analyzer program, the polyomavirus simian vacuolating virus 40 (SV40) [22] and Merkel Cell virus (MCV) [13] have been found to encode microRNA-like small RNAs, suggesting that VMir analyzer program is an effective tool for searching new viral miRNA-like small RNAs [52]. Therefore, we analyzed the genome of EBOV with the VMir software and obtained four pre-miRNAs located in the coding region of viral genome, indicating that the RNA secondary structures of EBOV genome might be processed into microRNA-like small RNAs [53, 54].

Infected cells have several signaling mechanisms to sense and respond to virus infection [55], for example, cross talk between different cellular pathways to modulate the expression and antiviral function of interferon (IFNs) with RIG-I-like receptor pathway and specific gene products. RIG-I-like receptor pathway and IFNs cytokines are important regulators of innate and adaptive immune responses [56]. Besides their antiviral role, they are potent regulators of cell growth and have immunomodulatory activity. INFs were activated after virus infection, probably through viral dsRNA and other viral gene products. The most intensely studied molecule in the RIG-I-like receptor pathway is the dsRNA-activated serine/threonine protein kinase (PKR). PKR was activated in the presence of cytoplasmic dsRNA, leading to the rapid phosphorylation of eukaryotic initiation factor eIF2 and subsequent inhibition of both host and viral mRNA [57, 58].

Although the bioinformatics prediction could be inaccurate, the bioinformatics prediction was potentially more selective and effective than experimental method. The target genes of viral genome-encoded microRNA-like small RNAs would help to develop an effective treatment for the EBOV infection.

5. Limitations

Due to the high mutation rate of reverse transcription in replication, EBOV presents numerous mutations over viral genome during host adaption, suggesting that the viral genome is not exactly the same among various EBOV strains. Thus, it is difficult to find microRNAs that are completely conserved among different viral strains due to genome mutations.

However, it is possible that some microRNA-like small RNAs are relatively conserved among diverse viral adapted hosts. Moreover, the expression pattern of viral microRNA-like small RNAs was highly unpredictable. Therefore, it might be difficult to validate the EBOV genome-encoded microRNA-like small RNAs using experimental method.

Acknowledgements

This work was supported by a grant from the State Key Laboratory of Pathogen and BioSecurity Program (No. SKLPBS1408 and No. SKLPBS1451).

Authors' contributions

Zhe Xu, Yuan Jin, and Xiaoping An characterized the materials, under the supervision of Yue Teng, Zhe Xu, and Dan Feng wrote the manuscript with further contributions from Jiangman Song and Yuan Jin analyzed the data. All authors reviewed the manuscript.

Conflict of interest

Competing financial interests and the authors declare no competing financial interests.

Author details

Yue Teng[1*], Zhe Xu[2], Jin Yuan[1], Xiaoping An[1], Jiangman Song[3] and Dan Feng[4]

*Address all correspondence to: yueteng@me.com; fddd@263.net

1 The State Key Laboratory of Pathogen and Biosecurity, Beijing Institute of Microbiology and Epidemiology, Beijing, China

2 Core Laboratory for Clinical Medical Research, Beijing Tiantan Hospital, Capital Medical University, Beijing, China

3 Department of Neurology, People's Hospital, Peking University, Beijing, China

4 Division of Standard Operational Management, Institute of Hospital Management, Chinese PLA General Hospital, Beijing, China

Yue Teng and Zhe Xu contributed equally to this work.

References

[1] Cenciarelli, O., Pietropaoli, S., Malizia, A., et al. Ebola virus disease 2013-2014 outbreak in west Africa: an analysis of the epidemic spread and response. *Int J Microbiol.* 2015, 769121 (2015).

[2] Ksiazek, T.G. Filoviruses: Marburg and Ebola. *Viral Infections of Humans.* 14, 337–350 (2014).

[3] World Health Organization. "Global Alert and Response (GAR): Situation Reports: Ebola Response Roadmap," 2015. Available at: http://www.who.int/csr/disease/ebola/situation-reports/en/.

[4] World Health Organization. "Ebola Situation Reports," 2014. Available at: http://apps.who.int/ebola/ebola-situation-reports.

[5] Frieden, T.R., Damon, I., Bell, B.P., Kenyon, T. and Nichol, S. Ebola 2014 – new challenges, new global response and responsibility. *N Eng J Med.* 371, 1117–1180 (2014).

[6] Walker, N.F., Whitty, C.J. Tackling emerging infections: clinical and public health lessons from the West African Ebola virus disease outbreak, 2014–2015. *Clin Med.* 15, 457–460 (2015).

[7] Alexander, K.A., Sanderson, C.E., Marathe, M., et al. What factors might have led to the emergence of Ebola in West Africa? *PLoS Negl Trop Dis.* 9(6), e0003652 (2015).

[8] Turner, C. Ebola virus disease: An emerging threat. *Nursing.* 44, 68–69 (2014).

[9] Kim, V. N., Han, J. and Siomi, M.C. Biogenesis of small RNAs in animals. *Nat Rev Mol Cell Biol.* 10, 128–139 (2009).

[10] Grundhoff, A. and Sullivan, C.S. Virus-encoded microRNAs. *Virology.* 411, 325–343 (2011).

[11] Brodersen P. and Voinnet, O. Revisiting the principles of microRNA target recognition and mode of action. *Nat Rev Mol Cell Biol.* 10, 141–148 (2009).

[12] Carthew, R.W. and Sontheimer, E.J. Origins and mechanisms of miRNAs and siRNAs. *Cell.* 136, 642–655 (2009).

[13] Seo, G.J., Chen, C.J. and Sullivan, C.S. Merkel cell polyomavirus encodes a microRNA with the ability to autoregulate viral gene expression. *Virology.* 383, 183–187 (2009).

[14] Pfeffer, S., et al. Identification of virus-encoded microRNAs. *Sicence.* 304, 734–736 (2004).

[15] Cullen, B.R. Viruses and microRNAs. *Nat Genet.* 38, S25–S30 (2006).

[16] Kincaid, R.P. and Sullivan, R.P. Virus-encoded microRNAls: an overview and a look to the future. *Plos Pathog.* 8, e10033018 (2012). DOI: 10.1371/journal.ppat.1003018.

[17] Lecellier, C.H., et al. A cellular microRNA mediates antiviral defense in human cells. *Science*. 308, 557–560 (2005).

[18] Walz, N., Christalla, T., Tessmer, U. and Grundhoff, A. A global analysis of evolutionary conservation among known and predicted gammaherpesvirus microRNAs. *J. Virol*. 84, 716–728 (2010).

[19] Sullivan, C.S., et al. SV40-encoded microRNAs regulate viral gene expression and reduce susceptibility to cytotoxic T cells. *Nature*. 435, 682–686 (2005).

[20] Samols, M.A., Hu, J., Skalsky, R.L. and Renne, R. Cloning and identification of a microRNA cluster within the latency-associated region of Kaposi's sarcoma-associated herpesvirus. *J. Virol*. 79, 9301–9305 (2005).

[21] Cui, C. Prediction and identification of herpes simplex virus 1-encoded microRNAs. *J. Virol*. 80, 5499–5508 (2006).

[22] Sullivan, C.S., Grundhoff, A.T., Tevethia, S., Pipas, J.M. and Ganem, D. SV40-encoded microRNAs regulate viral gene expression and reduce susceptibility to cytotoxic T cell. *Nature*. 435, 682–686 (2005).

[23] Cai, X., et al. Epstein-Barr virus microRNAs are evolutionarily conserved and differentially expressed. *PLoS Pathog*. 2, e23 (2006).

[24] Liang, H. Identification of Ebola virus microRNAs and their putative pathological function. *Sci China Life Sci*. 57, 973–981 (2014).

[25] Pfeffer, S., et al. Identification of microRNAs of the Herpesvirus family. *Nat. Methods*. 2, 269–276 (2005).

[26] Omoto, S., et al. HIV-1 nef suppression by virally encoded microRNA. *Retrovirology*. 1, 44 (2004).

[27] Bennasser, Y., et al. Evidence that HIV-1 encodes an siRNA and a suppressor of RNA silencing. *Immunity*. 22, 607–619 (2005).

[28] Rosewick, N. Deep sequencing reveals abundant noncanonical retroviral microRNAs in B-cell leukemia/lymphoma. *Proc. Natl. Acad. Sci. USA*. 110, 2306–2311 (2013).

[29] Gkirtzou, K., Tsamardinos, I., Tsakalides P. and Poirazi, P. MatureBayes: a probabilistic algorithm for identifying the mature miRNA within novel precursors. *Plos One*. 5, e11843 (2010). DOI: 10.1371/journal.pone.0011843.

[30] Katoh, K. and Standley, D.M. MAFFT multiple sequence alignment software version 7: improvements in performance and usability. *Mol Biol Evol*. 30, 772–780 (2013).

[31] Li, S.C., Shiau, C.K. and Lin, W.C. Vir-Mir db: prediction of viral microRNA candidate hairpins. *Nucleic Acids Res*. 36, 184–189 (2008).

[32] Jiang, P. MiPred: classification of real and pseudo microRNA precursors using random forest prediction model with combined features. *Nucleic Acids Res*. 35, 339–344 (2007).

[33] Sethupathy, P., Corda, B. and Hatziqeorqiou, A.G. TarBase: a comprehensive database of experimentally supported animal microRNA targets. *RNA*. 12, 192–197 (2006).

[34] Kanehisa, M. and Goto, S. KEGG: kyoto encyclopedia of genes and genomes. *Nucleic Acids Res*. 28, 27–30 (2000).

[35] Huang, D.W., Sherman, B.T. and Lempicki, R.A. Systematic and integrative analysis of large gene lists using DAVID bioinformatics resources. *Nat. Protoc*. 4, 44–57 (2009).

[36] Mi, H., Muruganujan, A. and Thomas, P.D. PANTHER in 2013: modeling the evolution of gene function, and other gene attributes, in the context of phylogenetic trees. *Nucleic Acids Res*. 41, 377–386 (2013).

[37] Mi, H., Muruganujan, A., Casaqrande, J.T. and Thomas, P.D. Large-scale gene function analysis with the PANTHER classification system. *Nat Protoc*. 8, 1551–1566 (2013).

[38] Franceschini, A., et al. STRING v9.1: protein-protein interaction networks, with increased coverage and integration. *Nucleic Acids Res*. 41, 808–815 (2013).

[39] Huang, D.W., Sherman, B.T. and Lempicki, R.A. Bioinformatics enrichment tools: paths toward the comprehensive functional analysis of large gene lists. *Nucleic Acids Res*. 37, 1–13 (2009).

[40] Bayarsaihan, D. Epigenetic mechanisms in inflammation. *J. Dent. Res*. 90, 9–17 (2011).

[41] Hayden, M.S., West, A.P. and Ghosh, S. NF-kappaB and the immune response. *Oncogene*. 25, 6758–6780 (2006).

[42] Bouwmeester, T. A physical and functional map of the human TNF-alpha/NF-kappa B signal transduction pathway. *Nat. Cell Biol*. 6, 97–105 (2004).

[43] Xu, W. Ebola virus VP24 targets a unique NLS binding site on karyopherin alpha 5 to selectively compete with nuclear import of phosphorylated STAT1. *Cell Host Microbe*. 16, 187–200 (2014).

[44] Kagoya, Y. Positive feedback between NF-kB and TNF-alpha promotes leukemia-initiating cell capacity. *J. Clin. Invest*. 124, 528–542 (2014).

[45] Lee, R.E., Walker, S.R., Savery, K., Frank, D.A. and Gaudet, S. Fold change of nuclear NF-kB determines TNF-induced transcription in single cells. *Mol. Cell*. 53, 867–879 (2014).

[46] Ramos, H.J. and Gale, M., Jr. RIG-I like receptors and their signaling crosstalk in the regulation of antiviral immunity. *Curr Opin Virol*. 1, 167–176 (2011).

[47] Loo, Y.M. and Gale, M., Jr. Immune signaling by RIG-I-like receptors. *Immunity*. 34, 680–692 (2011).

[48] Solis, M., et al. RIG-I-mediated antiviral signaling is inhibited in HIV-1 infection by a protease-mediated sequestration of RIG-I. *J Virol*. 85, 1224–1236 (2011).

[49] Pichlmair, A., et al. RIG-I-mediated antiviral responses to single-stranded RNA bearing 5'-phosphates. *Science*. 314, 997–1001 (2006).

[50] Gupta, A., et al. Anti-apoptotic function of a microRNA encoded by the HSV-1 latency-associated transcript. *Nature*. 442, 82–85 (2006).

[51] Satoh, T., et al. LGP2 is a positive regulator of RIG-I- and MDA5-mediated antiviral responses. *Proc Natl Acad Sci U S A*. 107, 1512–1517 (2010).

[52] Shi, J. Identification and validation of a novel microRNA-like molecule derived from a cytoplasmic RNA virus antigenome by bioinformatics and experimental approaches. *Virol. J*. 11, 121:1–121:14 (2014).

[53] Zuker, M. Mfold web server for nucleic acid folding and hybridization prediction. *Nucleic Acids Res*. 31, 3406–3415 (2003).

[54] Parisien, M. and Major, F. The MC-fold and MC-sym pipeline infers RNA structure from sequence data. *Nature*. 452, 51–55 (2008).

[55] Randall, R.E. and Goodbourn, S. Interferons and viruses: an interplay between induction, signalling, antiviral responses and virus countermeasures. *J. Gen. Virol*. 89, 1–47 (2008).

[56] Kaul, D., Ahlawat, A. and Gupta, S.D. HIV-1 genome-encoded HIV1-MIR-H1 impairs cellular responses to infection. *Mol. Cell Biochem*. 323, 143–148 (2009).

[57] Hussain, M. West Nile virus encodes a microRNA-like small RNA in the 3' untranslated region which up-regulates GATA4 mRNA and facilitates virus replication in mosquito cells. *Nucleic Acids Res*. 40, 2210–2223 (2012).

[58] Hussain, M., Taft, R.J. and Asgari, S. An insect virus-encoded microRNA regulates viral replication. *J. Virol*. 82, 9164–9170 (2008).

Section 3

Structure and Pathogenesis of Ebola Virus

Chapter 6

Roles of VP35, VP40 and VP24 Proteins of Ebola Virus in Pathogenic and Replication Mechanisms

Rahma Ait Hammou, Yassine Kasmi,
Khadija Khataby, Fatima Ezzahra Laasri,
Said Boughribil and My Mustapha Ennaji

Additional information is available at the end of the chapter

http://dx.doi.org/10.5772/63830

Abstract

Ebola epidemic is a fatal disease due to Ebola virus belonging to Filoviridae; currently the viral evolution caused more than 50% of death worldwide. Among the eight proteins of ZEBOV, there are four structural proteins VP35, VP40, VP24, and NP, which have important functions in the intercellular pathogenic mechanisms. The multi-functionality of Ebola's viral proteins allows the virus to reduce its protein number to ensure its proper functioning and keeping the compact structure of the virus. Therefore, the aim of this chapter is to study the mechanism of replication and the roles of VP30, VP35, NP, and L in this process. We provide as well to highlight the influence of the virus on the immune system and on the VP24.

Keywords: Ebola, VP35, VP40, VP24, pathogenic, replication, mechanisms, immune system

1. Introduction

Ebola is an acute viral disease that has appeared in 1976 in two simultaneous outbreaks, Nzara, South Sudan, and the other in Yambuku, Democratic Republic of Congo. The latter occurred in a village near the Ebola River, from which the disease takes its name "Ebola virus" which is an endemic virus of Africa. However, Ebola virus is a member of the filovirus family, characterized by multifunctional proteins. From the appointment of this family, these viruses are filamentous, and they present various forms such as (U), (L) and (6) under electronic microscope (**Figure 1**) [1]. Thus, viral propagation was due to the variant trips of populations through countries.

Although the multi-functionality of these proteins, each type has a specific role such as, GP protein that ensure important functions in the extracellular environment; otherwise, the VP35, VP40, and VP24 proteins have intracellular roles. eVP35 is usually used as symbol for "EBOLA's VP35 protein," one of the most important structural proteins of ZEBOV having diverse functions in pathogenesis mechanism and viral cycle [2]; it is an indispensable co-factor of replication transcription and an essential member of the replication complex. The virus has two other proteins, which play roles in immune response in intracellular stage.

Thus, the VP24 is a structural protein, that has the ability to internalize the cell nucleus, and known as a minor matrix protein and membrane-associated protein. Then, the latest protein "VP40" is known as a viral matrix protein, and it is the most abundant protein in Ebola's viral structure.

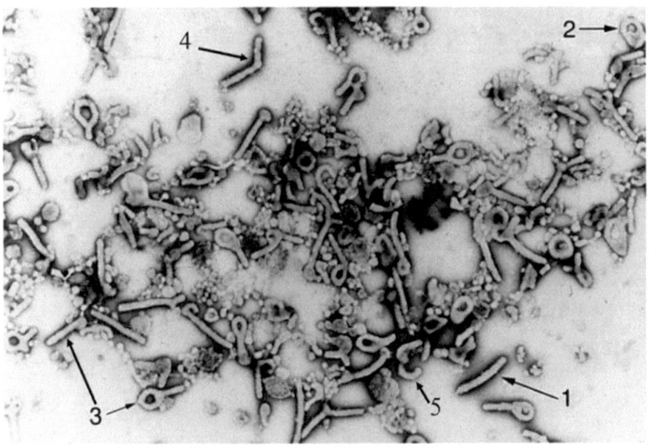

Figure 1. Marburg virus particles purified from the blood of infected guinea pigs, stained by negative contrast medium. Different forms of the virion are shown: 1, rod shaped; 2, ring shaped; 3, mace or (6); 4, (L) form, and 5, (U) form. Shaped '10.000' the virus was purified and concentrated by A, B, et al.; photo by E. Kandrushin, Center for Virology and Biotechnology "Vector," Koltsovo, Russia) [1].

Ebola is a zoonosis disease. The bats are the main natural reservoir of the virus, while also chimpanzee and some other animals could transmit EBOV virus to human. Transmission modes are diverse and not manageable: contact with fluids of infected persons, possibility of aerosol transmission [3, 4] and contact with infected animals [5]; here we must mention that the religious, cultural and traditional practices help the large propagation of virus among African population and that simple actions can limit the propagation of the virus. Epidemiological studies of WHO and CDC have shown that adults are more subjected to infection than children. Furthermore, Ebola virus can infect both men and women [6]. The virus has the ability to replicate in monocyte-derived dendritic cells without engendering an inflammatory response [7].

http://dx.doi.org/10.5772/63830

The transmission of Ebola virus to the human body is done by blood and spread in most cells, including vital organs, the infections in brain, liver and the heart disrupted the best functioning of these organs and thus occur as a direct result of death [8]. Time of replication *in vitro* is about 12 hours for Ebola virus on E6 cells [9].

2. How is the Filoviridae evolving?

We can find the answer of this question in phylogenic studies. Generally, the RNA viruses are characterized by the accumulation of many mutations during their evolution—these mutations are not predictable. Therefore, the Filoviridae is divided into genders that are distinct based on the numbers of mRNA encoding by GP gene. A study, demonstrate that the viral genome of this family is very similar. New phylogenetic analysis demonstrated that a few mutations in Reston genome can transfer the virus from non-Human pathogen to a Human pathogen, essentially in the VP24 gene: three VP24 SDPs (T131S, M136L, and Q139R) are likely to impair VP24 binding to human karyopherin alpha5 (KPNA5) and therefore inhibition of interferon signaling [10].

The human body mainly and the general superiors mammals consisting by several systems that achieve different functions to respond in the needs of body and assurance their life, among these systems, there are the immune system which has vital roles and performs important functions in the protection of the body and the eliminations of hazard. The immune system consists of several mechanisms and factors to ensure the proper functioning of the system; they can be subdivided into two under-system: innate immune and adaptive immune. The primary defenses against viral infections are the physical and chemical barriers: skin, pH, acidity, secretion, etc. First, the constituents of the innate response ensure the immune responses against viral agents, before request of the specific answer, another response corresponding to an innate response that is mediated by interferon (mainly interferon-γ), which promotes the activation of NK cells and CD 8 lymphocytes that recognize and destroy cells infected by the virus.

The aim of this chapter is to study the proteins VP35 and VP24 overlooking the immune system. In this chapter, we focus on the structures of those proteins, their roles, and their influence on immune responses.

3. Do the structural proteins have a role in the bending process of Filoviridae without breaking?

More than 50% of the virions grown in cells are polyploidy. Most families of viruses have a single copy of the genome by particle. However, polyploidy is relatively rare in the viral world [11]. Among these families is the *Paramyxoviridae* [12]; so the first assumption is that the Filoviridae are of polyploidy. In addition, the second is the flexibility of the nucleocapsid (RNA, VP30, VP35, N, and L) with the intervention of the VP24 protein [13].

4. Structural and genomic information

The genome of the Filoviridae is rather similar, with seven genes that encoding for the seven proteins or eighth for Ebola. The genes contain the respective open reading frame (ORF) flanked by unusually long non-translated sequences, ranging from 57 to 684 nucleotides [14]. The VP24 protein is expressed by the region 9886–11497, and the region 11498–11501 is an intergenic region, which ensures essential roles for the virus: It is immunosuppressive [15] that allows the virus to control the innate immune system [16]; it binds directly with STAT1 causing antagonize interferon [17]. VP40 has various roles; unmodified polypeptide may assemble into different structures for different functions [18]. The rates of conservation of Filoviridae proteins are 33% for VP35, 27% for VP40, 34% for GP, 33% for VP30, and 37% for VP 24. The board 3′ and 5′ regions ensures important functions in replication, transcription of the genome, and its control.VP35 gene advance by a conserved transcription start and stop signals, "CUACUU-CUAAUU" for start and "UAAUUCU" as stop transcription signal. However, the coding start of VP40 is "CUACUUCUAAUU," and then signal stop is "UAAUUCU." For the viral protein 24 (VP24), the signal start "CUACUUCUAAUU" is sited in position 9886–9897 from Genome's Ebola. However, the VP24 has two stop signals "UAAUUCU" [19]. The genome of EBOV is schematically shown in **Figure 2**.

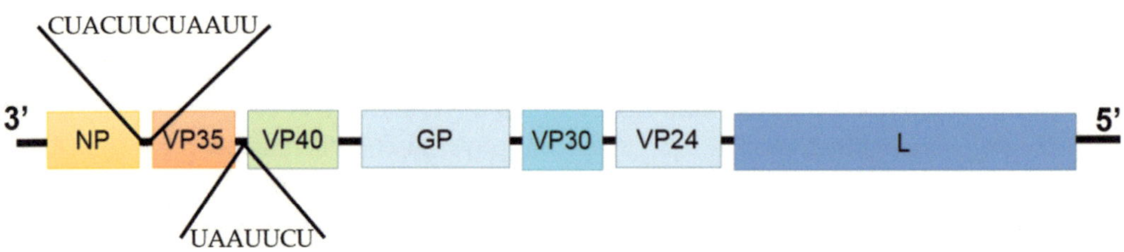

Figure 2. The full-length genome of Ebola is about 19,000 nucleotide, where L gene coding for the RNA polymerase, it is the length gene and more conserved gene in the Filoviridae, then the VP40 is the more polymorphism gene.

The VP35 gene located among the position 3032 and 4407 of Ebola genome, coding for alone mRNA with same length, though the regulatory region is located at the nucleotide 3032 and 3048 "CUACUUCUAAUU" which is a transcription start signal. For the VP40, it is sited at the 4390th nucleotide and 5894th, with one mRNA at the same length, and thus the start signal is on position 4390th to 4401th; besides region 4397–4407and 5883–5894 in genome are two poly-adenine signal sequences [20].

A single mutation in the central basic patch residue R322 or end-cap residue F239 to alanine capable to disrupt the dsRNA binding and alters VP35 inhibitor of RIG1 [21, 22]. These mutants retain modest inhibitory activity relative to the empty vector control. Thus, they exhibited reduced suppression of SeV-induced IFNα/β production [23].

The dsRNA-binding cluster is centered on Arg-312, a highly conserved residue required for IFN inhibition. Importantly, the stability of the β-sheet subdomain structure of VP35 requests an interaction between the side chains of Pro-315, Pro-318, and Lys-339 residues and conserved

http://dx.doi.org/10.5772/63830

Trp-324, as well as the Ile-340 residue, which make bond with Phe-239, Leu-242, and Ile-278 (**Figure 3**). These residues are highly conserved in Ebola genome, and that demonstrates the importance of these residues in the stability and the good functioning of the VP35 protein [24].

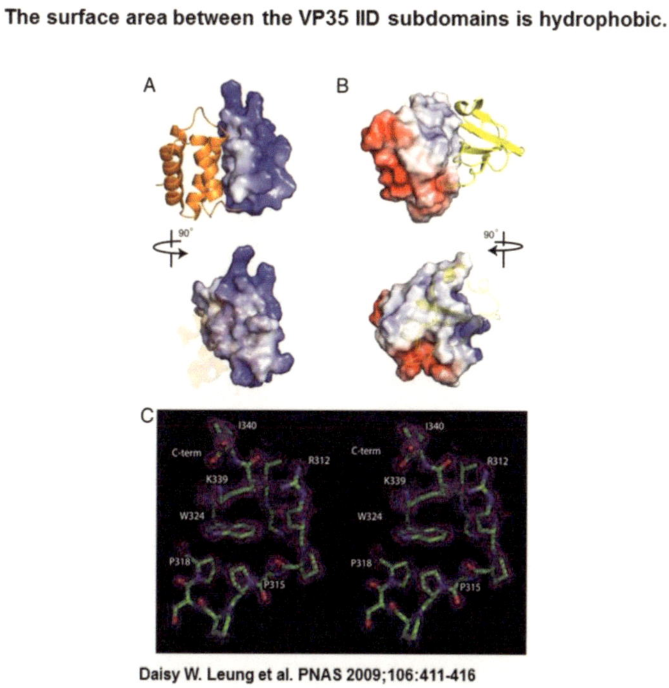

Figure 3. The surface area between the VP35 IID subdomains is hydrophobic. (A and B) Electrostatic representations of the inter-subdomain interaction surface for the α-helical subdomain (A) and the β-sheet subdomain (B) reveal hydrophobic surfaces buried between the two subdomains. Red, white, and blue represent negative, neutral, and positive electrostatic potentials, respectively (range -5 to +5 kT). (C) Stereographic image showing the Trp-324 side chain making important hydrophobic contacts with residues in β4 strand, α5 helix, and PPII [24].

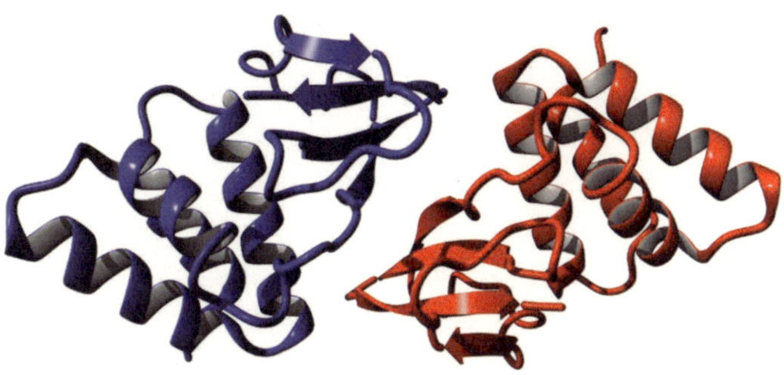

Figure 4. A crystal structure of VP35 from RCSB databank number 4IBB, obtunded X-RAY DIFFRACTION method with a resolution of 1.84 Å R-Value Free: 0.233 and R-Value Work: 0.177. The VP35 has two sub units with 4 β-sheets and 4 α helices [25].

The work of Mateo et al. 2010 [25] has dismiss that the amino acids in position 1–20 of VP24 are not important in the functioning of VP24 to inhibit IFN-β-induced gene expression. However, mutations in position 44 influence on the function of VP24 and have a critical role in the inhibition of IFN-β-induced gene expression. However, residues 142–146 are important to inhibit ISG54 activation by IFN-β. Therefore, mutations at residues 142–146 are able to increase the expression of ISG54 reporter up to 90%, thus drastically reducing VP24 activity [26]. Structure of VP24 dimer is shown as **Figure 5**.

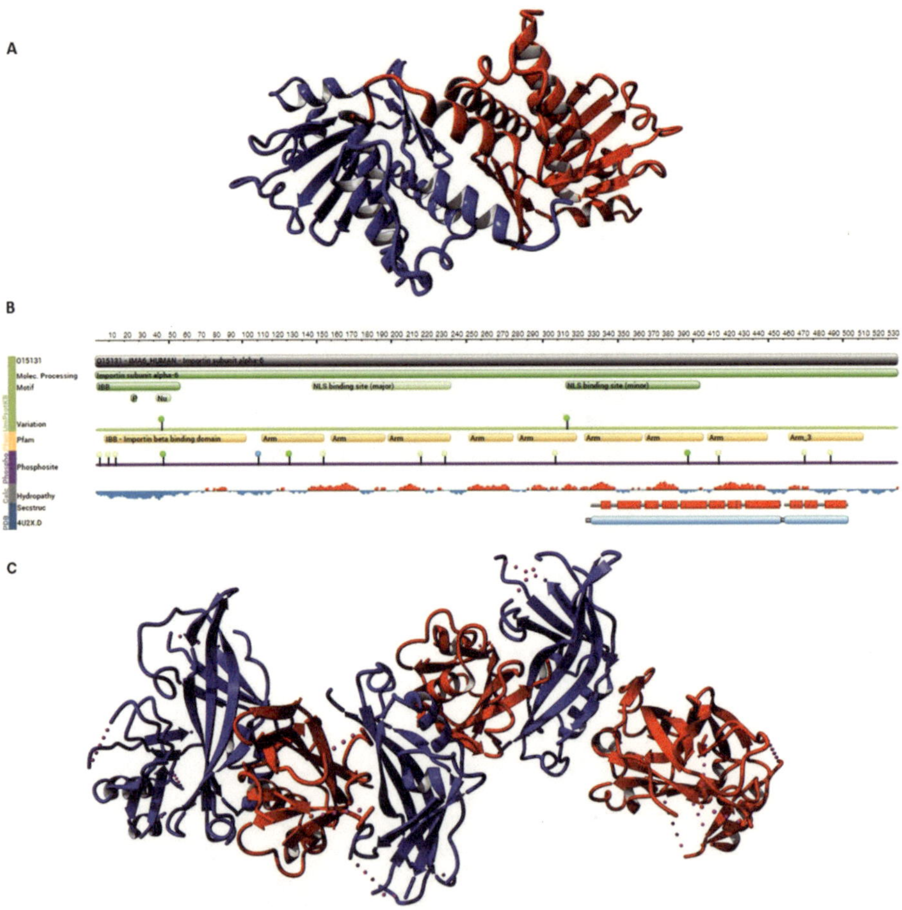

Figure 5. *(A) Ebola virus VP24 structure (4M0Q) from RCSB with (B) resolution of 1.92 Å, then b. is Protein Feature View—UniProtKB AC: Q05322. The VP35 has two subunits with 8 β-sheet and 5 α helices. The length amino acids chain is 251AA [27]. (C) Crystal image of VP40 Hexamer [29].*

Residues 213–326 are essential for VP40 to associate with liposomes; 309–317 has a critical role in the associated with the DSM fraction; the truncation of 18 C-terminal residues resulted in predominantly oligomeric protein that mainly associated with the DSM fraction [28].

http://dx.doi.org/10.5772/63830

5. Ebola virus replication

The replication process in the mono-nonsense-negative genome is almost similar; the first step is the transfer from negative sense genome to positive sense genome. The positive sense genome (call also anti-genome or complementary genome) is the complement RNA sequence, direct sense of transcription. From the positive sense genome, two processes are done: the first is replication and getting the negative sense genome for formation of new virion, the second calling the cellular ribosome for the translate process for making new viral proteins (**Figure 6**).

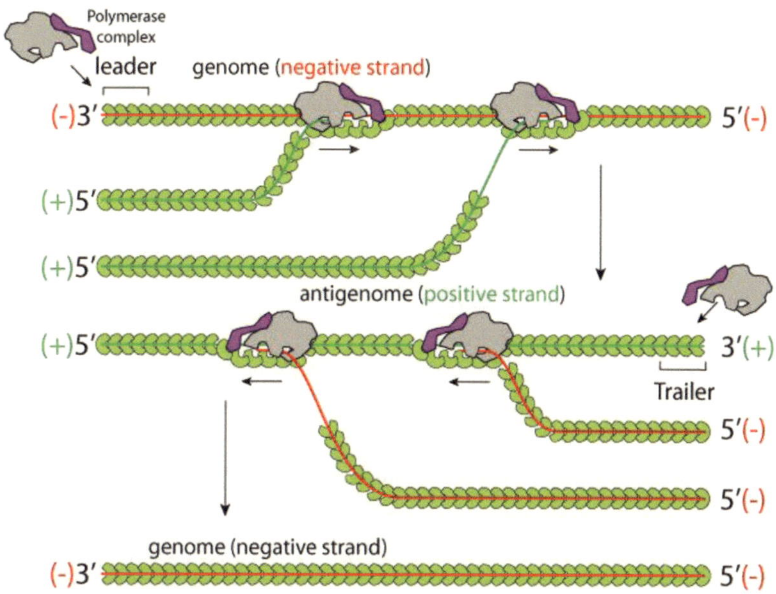

Figure 6. The transcription and replication process, the virus pass from negative sense to positive and from positive to negative sense [30].

The Ebola virus life cycle can be spread over following stages: the first stages are adsorption and penetration in the cell, followed by de-capsulation, transfer genome from negative to positive, primary and syntheses transcription of functional proteins, second transcription replication and assembly of virus.

For Ebola virus, after the liberation of VP30, VP35, L, VP40, and VP24 with the genome in cytoplasm, the first step is the formation of replication complex composed by L (RNA polymerase), VP35, NP, and VP30. The VP30 is an indispensable co-factor of transcription, even the VP30 is part of this complex as transcription activator, and it is a highly phosphorylated [31]. The L is the polymerase protein of EBOV; it is the large protein in genome and the most conserved protein among Filoviridae. In addition to the transcription and replication functions, it can connect the VP35 and NP where NP-RNA helices associate with VP35. Ebola virus VP35 is essential for nucleocapsid formation, together with NP and VP24 [32].

The initiation of transcription requires a VP30 signal, and this signal takes place after attachment of zinc molecule in zinc-binding Cys3-His motif comprising amino acids 68–95 [33]. The phosphorylation site is a conserved site, where a simple mutation can get negative effects on the incorporation of VP30 with the other viral particles and therefore affect the efficiency of the recovery of the viruses [31]. The frequency of transcription of an mRNA is different following the position of the gene in genome, the genes proximal to 3′ are more translated than those in 5′, thanks to the second mRNA produce and that contains essentially [34]. The interagency regions ensure a role in the control and the regulation of replication and transcription of virus [35].

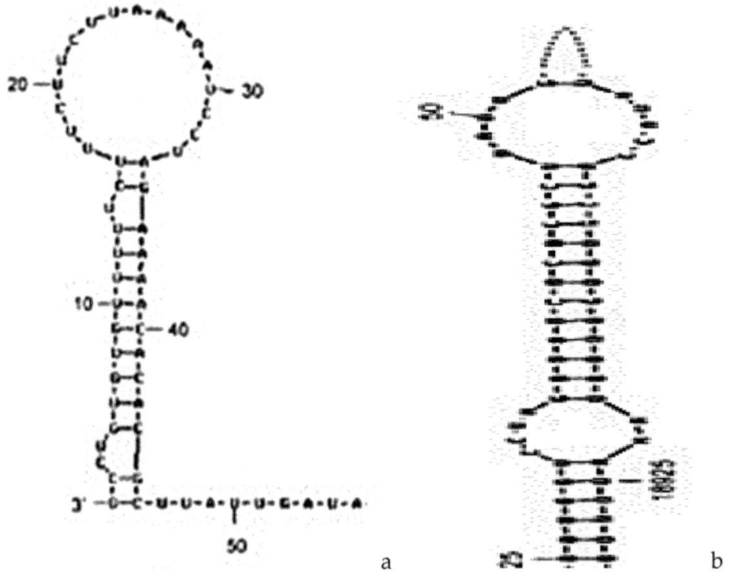

Figure 7. Two secondary structures predicted of ZEBOV genomic RNA. The interactions made by (a) a hairpin structure (b) and panhandle structure format [33].

The RNA bonds with the complex of VP35-NP-L to initiate the replication and transcription of viral genome. Translation of viral protein is ensured by liberation ribosome in cytoplasm. The replication mechanism is not manageable enough; however, there are estimates of the true mechanism of replication.

Weik and their collaborators in 2005 [36] demonstrate that the nucleotides 5–44 of the EBOV leader are involved in RNA secondary-structure formation; the alteration of 36 nucleotides spanning the region 55–90 did not affect replication. However, when the random sequence was elongated by four additional nucleotides, replication activity could not be detected. Bipartite promoters localized in 3′ of gene, and then the second signal is in the beginning of the next gene; it is a succession of eight UN5 hexamer repeats (**Figure 7**) [36], other research shows that EBOV NP is inactive in Marburg the vice-versa, and this suggests that they present a specific motifs by the complex of replication for each gender. The region of the EBOV

http://dx.doi.org/10.5772/63830

promoter start signal of the NP gene (12 nucleotides) and the following 13 nucleotides has been shown to form a stem-loop structure, which is involved in regulation of VP30-dependent transcription [1]. Other results of Brauburger et al. 2014 [37] reflect fundamental differences in the control of polymerase behavior by cis-acting sequences between viruses with conserved and variable gene borders and suggest an important role of conserved IRs in transcription regulation, while the function of variable IRs remains less clear.

6. Ebola and immune system

The Ebola virus has the ability to flare the immune system by several modes. Furthermore, the virus uses the immune system as tools to fix and internalize in cell, thanks to the link between GP and the antibody as demonstrated in the chapter of Glycoprotein. Mahanty and others [38] illustrate in the **Figure 8** some immune evasion tools [38].

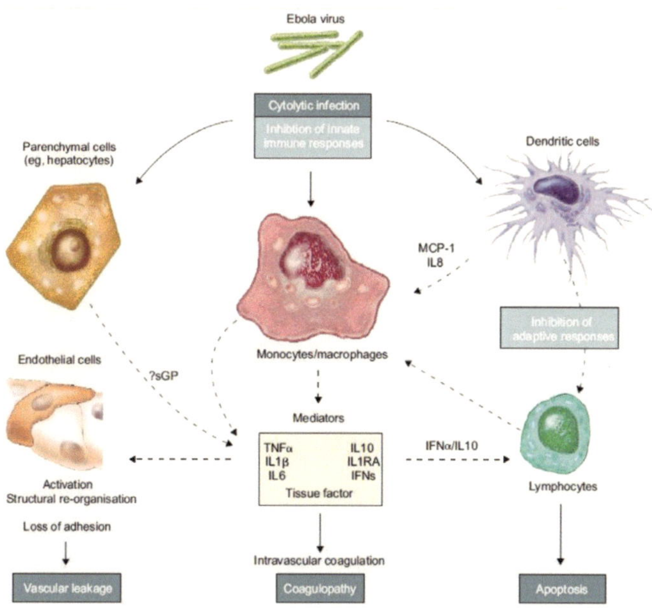

Figure 8. A model of the pathogenesis of filoviral hemorrhagic fever, based on studies of Zaire Ebola virus infection. Infection causes lysis of monocytes/macrophages, dendritic cells, and hepatocytes and suppresses innate immune responses in these cells, aiding further dissemination. Direct injury to infected cells is accompanied by indirect effects that are mediated by pro-inflammatory and anti-inflammatory effector molecules, including interleukin 1 (IL1), interleukin 6 (IL6), TNF, interleukin 10 (IL10), and type I interferons (IFN). The severe illness results from the combined effects of widespread viral cytolysis and massive release of pro-inflammatory mediators. Pro-inflammatory cytokines and chemokines are also produced by activated endothelial cells, resulting in a feedback loop to the monocytes/macrophages. Lymphocyte apoptosis is also apparently brought about through effects of pro-inflammatory mediators; it may contribute to immunosuppression by weakening adaptive immune responses. The cell-surface expression of tissue factor by virus-infected monocytes/macrophages induces disseminated intravascular coagulation. MCP monocyte chemoattractant protein; IL1RA interleukin-1 receptor antagonist [39].

Here, we discuss the intracellular mechanism to escape the immune system via structural proteins and their roles in inhibition of the interferon's expression (**Figure 9**).

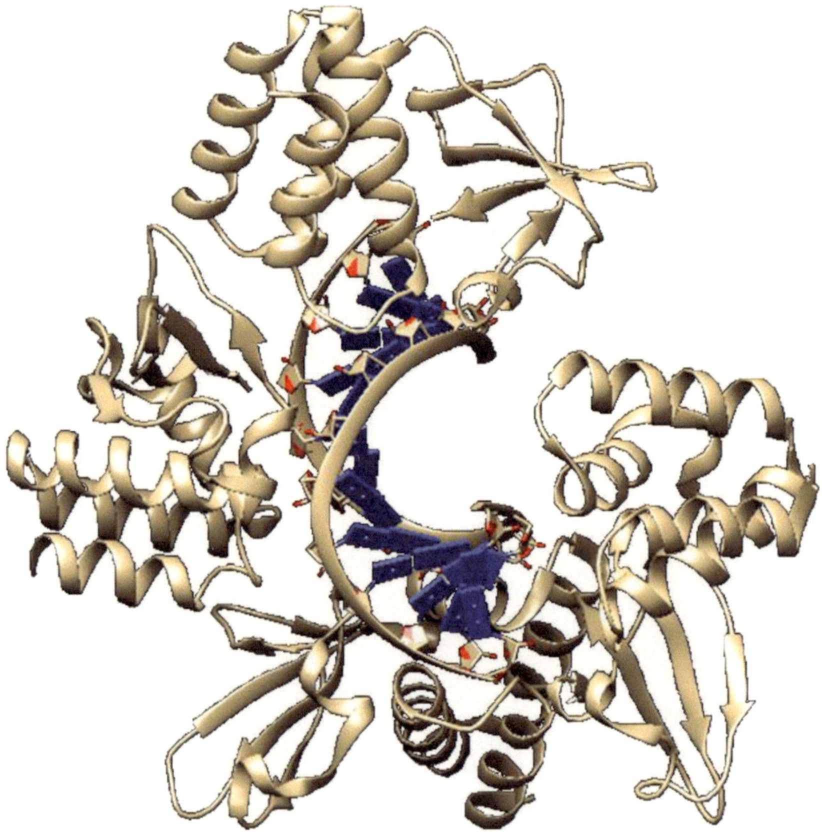

Figure 9. The crystal structure of VP35 bond to dsRNA [41].

The VP35 implicated in modulation of the host immune response. Studies show that the region C-terminal-binding site with the dsRNA in VP 35 is being demonstrated as responsible of antagonism region's interferon and immune evasion. The VP35 bond specifically with specifically with poly(rI) poly(rC), poly(rA), poly(rU) [39].

The VP35 through PACT has the ability to inhibit the retinoic acid inducible Gene-I (RIG-I) to bind with the dsRNA, and this action inhibits the transfer of hazardous signal to the interferon promoter simulator I by RIG-I in first time. Therefore, if the signal has transferred by the RIG-I, the VP35 binds to the Tank-binding kinase-1 interferon kinases (TBK-1/IKKε) and inhibiting the phosphorylation of IRF-3/7 [40–43]. Consequently, the translocation nucleus of signal and the expression of INF-β will be inhibited (**Figure 10**). More recent study suggests that other filoviral proteins, including EBOV VP30 and VP40, also counter the RNAi pathway [44].

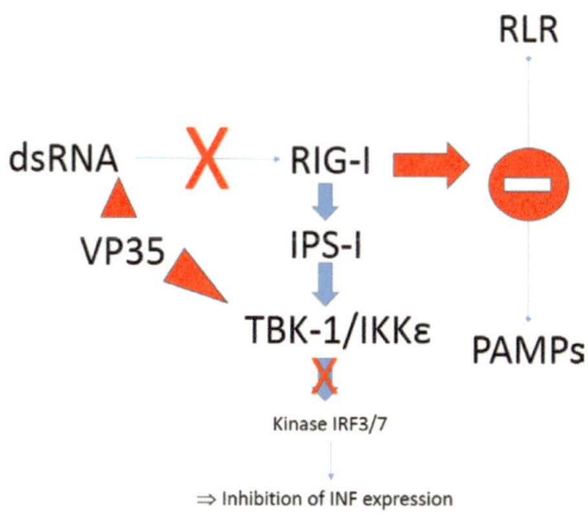

Figure 10. The inhibition of the recognition of PAMPs by the RLR, due to the inhibition of RIG-1 by bonding of VP35 to dsRNA through the CBP.

However, Luther and their collaborator's in 2013 [45] had shown that the PACT also implicated in inhibition of RIG-I. Other studies shown that the mVP35 and eVP35 effects differently the RIG-I, ebolaVP35 blocked the RIG-I then Marburg VP35 decreased the affinity and the activity of RIG-I [46].

The same context of INF-β's inhibition, the VP40 interacted with the Janus kinase/tyrosine kinase II (JAK I/TRK II) for block their phosphorylation and as results, inhibition of the activation of STAT heterodimer kinase require the phosphorylation of JAK-I/TRK II [47, 48].

In the other hand, VP24 bonds with Karyopherin-α by the residues in activation of sites 26–50 and 142–146 and they are demonstrated to be the most important residues for this activity (**Figure 11**) [46].

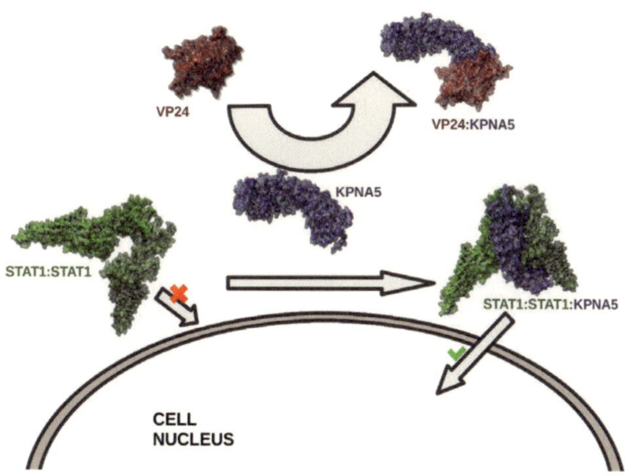

Figure 11. The binding between VP24 and KPNA5, *and* this link in the active site of STAT homodimer. It prevents the adhesion of the SATA homodimer phosphorylated and thus lack the protein's ability to enter the cell nucleus.

7. Inhibition strategies of Ebola virus

The involvement of VP35 in diverse parts of the infection (replication, inhibition of RIG1, TAK, and inhibition of interferon) made it a principal target of several medicines to inhibit it. Thus, all the Ebola proteins are crystallized and available in databases as RCSB, addition to the full-length genome sequenced is available in NCBI databases make research and information about the virus more accessible (**Figure 12**).

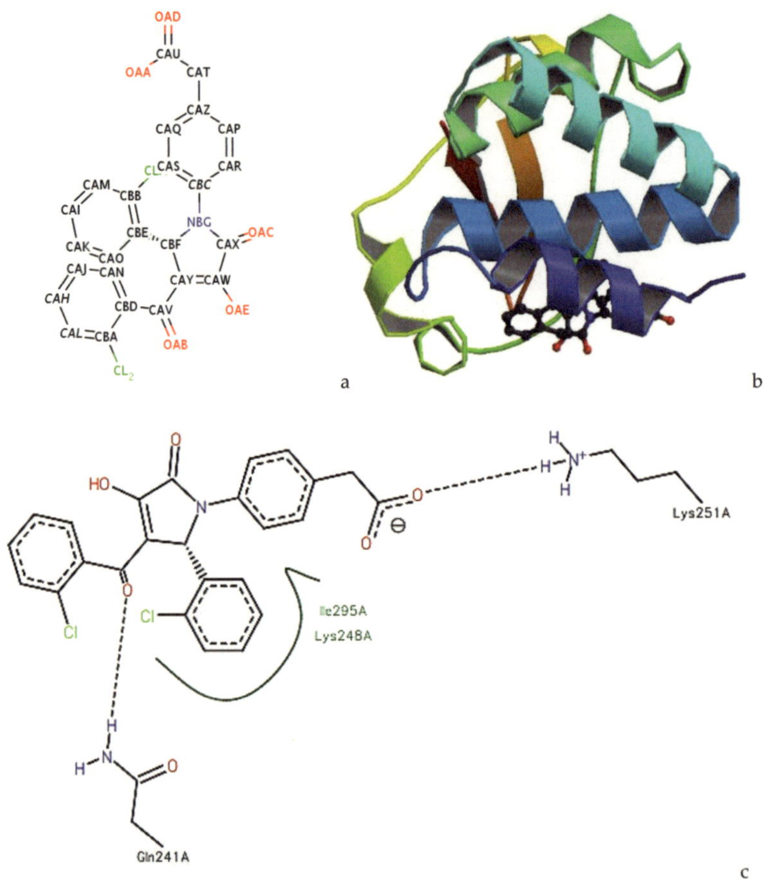

Figure 12. In silico-derived small molecules, it binds the filovirus *VP35* protein and inhibit its polymerase cofactor activity. (a) {4-[(2R)-3-(2-chlorobenzoyl)-2-(2-chlorophenyl)-4-hydroxy-5-oxo-2,5-dihydro-1H-pyrrol-1-yl]phenyl}acetic acid. (b) *3D with ligand.* (c) The *pharmacophore map of ligand in the active site of VP35* [49].

8. Conclusions

The light of the above discussion results, the Filoviridae genome coding seven proteins, with the exception of Ebola virus that coded for the eight proteins, including the GP gene which coded for secretory glycoproteins, membrane glycoproteins, and thus it is subdivided into subunits called as GP1 and GP2. However, the sGP has not the membrane region. The Ebola genome contains six interagency regions, having functions in regulation of transcription of genes and the CAP-polyA to protect the mRNA. Those regions contain a RNA 2D confirmation boots. The immune evasion processes in Filoviridae generally, and essentially for Ebola virus based on two complementary process; one intercellular by GP and second intracellular where the roles remarkable of VP35 by inhibition of RIG-I and INF-3, therefore, the roles of VP40 and VP24 inhibition of INF-β signal.

Acknowledgements

The authors would like to thank the ministry of higher education, University Hassan II of Casablanca, Faculty of Sciences and Technics and the Laboratory of Virology, Microbiology, Quality and Biotechnologies/Ecotoxicology and Biodiversity.

Author details

Rahma Ait Hammou, Yassine Kasmi, Khadija Khataby, Fatima Ezzahra Laasri, Said Boughribil and My Mustapha Ennaji*

*Address all correspondence to: m.ennaji@yahoo.fr

Laboratory of Virology, Microbiology, Quality and Biotechnologies/Eco-toxicology and Biodiversity, Team of Virology, Oncology and Medical Biotechnologies, Faculty of Sciences and Techniques, University Hassan II of Casablanca, Mohammedia, Morocco

Rahma Ait Hammou and Yassine Kasmi contributed equally to this work.

References

[1] Beer, B., Kurth, R., & Bukreyev, A. (1999). Characteristics of filoviridae: Marburg and Ebola viruses. Naturwissenschaften, 86(1):8–17.

[2] Bagherani, N., Smoller, B. R., Kannangara, A. P., Gianfaldoni, S., Wang, X., & Goren, A. (2015). An Overview on Ebola. Department of Dermatology, University of Rome, Italy, 2, 64–73.

[3] Jahrling, P. B., Geisbert, T. W., Dalgard, D.W., et al. (1990). Preliminary report: isolation of Ebola virus from monkeys imported to USA. LANCET, 335:502–5.

[4] Centers for Disease Control. (1990). Update: Ebola-related filovirus infection in nonhuman primates and interim guidelines for handling nonhuman primates during

transit and quarantine. MMWR, 39:22–4, 29–30. http://www.cdc.gov/mmwr/preview/mmwrhtml/00001538.htm consulted in 4th, 2016, April.

[5] Leroy, E. M., Rouquet, P., Formenty, P., Souquiere, S., Kilbourne, A., Froment, J. M., & Zaki, S. R. (2004). Multiple Ebola virus transmission events and rapid decline of central African wildlife. Science, 303(5656):387–390.

[6] http://www.who.int/mediacentre/news/releases/2014/ebola-study/en/

[7] Bosio, C. M., Aman, M. J., Grogan, C., Hogan, R., Ruthel, G., Negley, D., & Schmaljohn, A. (2003). Ebola and Marburg viruses replicate in monocyte-derived dendritic cells without inducing the production of cytokines and full maturation. Journal of Infectious Diseases, 188(11):1630–1638.

[8] Falasca, L., Agrati, C., Petrosillo, N., Di Caro, A., Capobianchi, M. R., Ippolito, G., & Piacentini, M. (2015). Molecular mechanisms of Ebola virus pathogenesis: focus on cell death. Cell Death & Differentiation, 22(8):1250–1259.

[9] Sanchez, A., & Kiley, M. P. (1987). Identification and analysis of Ebola virus messenger RNA. Virology, 157(2):414–420.

[10] Pappalardo, M., Juliá, M., Howard, M. J., Rossman, J. S., Michaelis, M., Wass, M. N. (2016). Conserved differences in protein sequence determine the human pathogenicity of Ebola viruses. Scientific Reports, 6.

[11] Luque, D. et al. (2009). Infectious bursal disease virus is an icosahedral polyploid dsRNA virus. Proceedings of the National Academy of Sciences USA, 106:2148–2152.

[12] Rager, M. et al. (2002). Polyploid measles virus with hexameric genome length. EMBO Journal. 21:2364–2372

[13] Booth, T. F., Rabb, M. J., & Beniac, D. R. (2013). How do filovirus filaments bend without breaking? Trends in Microbiology, 21(11):583–593.

[14] Mühlberger, E. (2007). Filovirus replication and transcription Future Virology, 2 (2), 205–215 DOI: 10.2217/17460794.2.2.205

[15] Zhanga, A. P. P., Bornholdta, Z. A., Abelsona, D. M., & Saphire, E. O. (2014) "Crystal structure of Marburg virus VP24", Published ahead of print 26 February 2014. Journal of Virology, 88(10):5859–5863. W. I. Sundquist, Editor. doi:10.1128/JVI.03565–13

[16] Mateo, M. (2010). Etude du role de la proteine VP24 dans la replication, la pathogenicite et l'adaptation du virus Ebola (Doctoral dissertation, Lyon, École normale superieure (Sciences)).

[17] Zhang, A. P. P., Bornholdt, Z. A., Liu, T., Abelson, D. M., Lee, D. E., Sheng L. I., Virgil, L., Woods, J. R., Saphire, E. O. (2012) "The Ebola virus interferon antagonist VP24 directly binds STAT1 and has a novel, pyramidal fold". Plos Pathogens, 8(2):E1002550. Published online Feb 23, 2012. doi:10.1371/journal.ppat.1002550 PMCID: PMC3285596, Félix A. Rey, Editor.

[18] Bornholdt, Z. A., Noda, T., Abelson, D. M., Halfmann, P., Wood, M. R., Kawaoka, Y., & Saphire, E. O. (2013) "Structural rearrangement of Ebola virus VP40 begets multiple functions in the virus life cycle". Cell, 154:763–774. Elsevier Inc. doi:10.1016/j.cell.2013.07.015

[19] Lee, J. E., Fusco, M. L., Hessell, A. J., Oswald, W. B., Burton, D. R., & Saphire, E. O. (2008). Structure of the Ebola virus glycoprotein bound to an antibody from a human survivor. Nature, 454(7201):177–182.

[20] Kugelman, J. R., Rossi, C. A., Wiley, M. R., Ladner, J. T., Nagle, E. R., Pfeffer, B. P., & Palacios, G. (2016). Informing the historical record of experimental nonhuman primate infections with Ebola virus: genomic characterization of USAMRIID Ebola virus/H. Sapiens-tc/COD/1995/Kikwit-9510621 challenge stock "R4368" and its replacement "R4415". Plos One, 11(3):E0150919.

[21] Prins, K. C., Delpeut, S., Leung, D. W., Reynard, O., Volchkova, V. A., Reid, S. P., Ramanan, P., Cardenas, W. B., Amarasinghe, G. K., Volchkov, V. E., Basler, C. F. (2010). Mutations abrogating VP35 interaction with double-stranded RNA render Ebola virus a virulent in guinea pigs. Journal of Virology. 84:3004–3015. doi:10.1128/JVI.02459-09

[22] Luthra, P., Ramanan, P., Mire, C. E., Weisend, C., Tsuda, Y., Yen, B., Liu, G., Leung, D. W., Geisbert, T. W., Ebihara, H., Amarasinghe, G. K., Basler, C. F. (2013). Mutual antagonism between the Ebola virus VP35 Protein and the RIG-I activator pact determines infection outcome. Cell Host Microbe, 14:74–84. doi:10.1016/J.CHOM.2013.06.010

[23] Yen, B., Mulder, L. C., Martinez, O., & Basler, C. F. (2014). Molecular basis for Ebola virus VP35 suppression of human dendritic cell maturation. Journal of Virology, 88(21):12500–12510.

[24] Leung, D. W., Ginder, N. D., Fulton, D. B., Nix, J., Basler, C. F., Honzatko, R. B., & Amarasinghe, G. K. (2009). Structure of the Ebola VP35 interferon inhibitory domain. Proceedings of the National Academy of Sciences, 106(2):411–416.

[25] Brown, C. S., Lee, M. S., Leung, D. W., Wang, T., Xu, W., Luthra, P., & Borek, D. M. (2014). In silico derived small molecules bind the filovirus VP35 protein and inhibit its polymerase cofactor activity. Journal of Molecular Biology, 426(10):2045–2058.

[26] Mateo, M., Leung, L. W., Basler, C. F., & Volchkov, V. E. (2010). Ebola virus VP24 binding to karyopherins is required for inhibition of interferon signaling. Journal of Virology, 84(2):1169–1175.

[27] From RSCB Data Base Consulted in 4th, 2016 April.

[28] Panchal, R. G., Ruthel, G., Kenny, T. A., Kallstrom, G. H., Lane, D., Badie, S. S., & Aman, M. J. (2003). In vivo oligomerization and raft localization of Ebola virus protein VP40 during vesicular budding. Proceedings of the National Academy of Sciences, 100(26):15936–15941.

[29] Bornholdt, Z. A., Noda, T., Abelson, D. M., Halfmann, P., Wood, M. R., Kawaoka, Y., & Saphire, E. O. (2013). Structural rearrangement of Ebola virus VP40 begets multiple functions in the virus life cycle. Cell, 154(4):763–774.

[30] http://viralzone.expasy.org/all_by_protein/1096.html consulted 4th, 2016, April. http://viralzone.expasy.org/all_by_protein/1096.html

[31] Martínez, M. J., Biedenkopf, N., Volchkova, V., Hartlieb, B., Alazard-Dany, N., Reynard, O., & Volchkov, V. (2008). Role of Ebola virus VP30 in transcription reinitiation. Journal of Virology, 82(24):12569–12573.

[32] Noda, T., Kolesnikova, L., Becker, S., & Kawaoka, Y. (2011). The importance of the NP:VP35 ratio in Ebola virus nucleocapsid formation. Journal of Infectious Diseases, 204(Suppl 3):S878–S883.

[33] Modrof, J., Becker, S., & Mühlberger, E. (2003). Ebola virus transcription activator VP30 is a zinc-binding protein. Journal of Virology, 77(5):3334–3338.

[34] Mühlberger, E., Lötfering, B., Klenk, H. D., & Becker, S. (1998). Three of the four nucleocapsid proteins of Marburg virus, NP, VP35, and L, are sufficient to mediate replication and transcription of Marburg virus-specific monocistronic minigenomes. Journal of Virology, 72(11):8756–8764.

[35] Biedenkopf, N. (2012). Die phosphorylierung des Ebolavirus VP30 reguliert die virale transkription und replikation.

[36] Weik, M., Enterlein, S., Schlenz, K., & Mühlberger, E. (2005). The Ebola virus genomic replication promoter is bipartite and follows the rule of six. Journal of Virology, 79(16): 10660–10671.

[37] Weik, M., Modrof, J., Klenk, H. D., Becker, S., & Mühlberger, E. (2002). Ebola virus VP30-mediated transcription is regulated by RNA secondary structure formation. Journal of Virology, 76:8532–8539.

[38] Brauburger, K., Boehmann, Y., Tsuda, Y., Hoenen, T., Olejnik, J., Schümann, M., & Mühlberger, E. (2014). Analysis of the highly diverse gene borders in Ebola virus reveals a distinct mechanism of transcriptional regulation. Journal of Virology, 88(21): 12558–12571.

[39] Mahanty, S., Bray, M. (2004). Pathogenesis of filoviral haemorrhagic fevers. The Lancet Infectious Diseases, 4(8):487–498.

[40] Cárdenas, W. B., Loo, Y. M., Gale, M., Hartman, A. L., Kimberlin, C. R., Martínez-Sobrido, L., & Basler, C. F. (2006). Ebola virus VP35 protein binds double-stranded RNA and inhibits alpha/beta interferon production induced by RIG-I signaling. Journal of Virology, 80(11):5168–5178.

[41] Prins, K. C., Cardenas, W. B., Basler, C. F. (2009) Ebola virus protein VP35 impairs the function of interferon regulatory factor-activating kinases IKKε and TBK-1. Journal of Virology, 83:3069–3077.

[42] Bale, S., Julien, J. P., Bornholdt, Z. A., Krois, A. S., Wilson, I. A., Saphire, E. O. (2013). Ebola virus VP35 coats the backbone of double-stranded RNA for interferon antagonism. Journal of Virology, 87:10385–10388.

[43] Bale, S., Julien, J. P., Bornholdt, Z. A., Kimberlin, C. R., Halfmann, P., Zandonatti, M. A., Kunert, J., Kroon, G. J., Kawaoka, Y., Macrae, I. J., Wilson, I. A., Saphire, E. O. (2012). Marburg virus VP35 can both fully coat the backbone and cap the ends of dsRNA for interferon antagonism. Plos Pathogens, 8:E1002916.

[44] Leung, D. W., Ginder, N. D., Fulton, D. B., Nix, J., Basler, C. F., Honzatko, R. B., Amarasinghe, G. K. (2009). Structure of the Ebola VP35 interferon inhibitory domain. Proceedings of the National Academy of Sciences USA, 106:411–416.

[45] Leung, D. W., Prins, K. C., Borek, D. M., Farahbakhsh, M., Tufariello, J. M., Ramanan, P., Nix, J. C., Helgeson, L. A., Otwinowski, Z., Honzatko, R. B., Basler, C. F., Amara Singhe, G. K. (2010). Structural basis for dsRNA recognition and interferon antagonism by Ebola VP35. Nature Structural & Molecular Biology, 17:165–172.

[46] Ramanan, P., Shabman, R. S., Brown, C. S., Amarasinghe, G. K., Basler, C. F., & Leung, D. W. (2011). Filoviral immune evasion mechanisms. Viruses, 3(9):1634–1649.

[47] Luthra, P., Ramanan, P., Mire, C. E., Weisend, C., Tsuda, Y., Yen, B., Liu, G., Leung, D. W., Geisbert, T. W., Ebihara, H., Amarasinghe, G. K., Basler, C. F. (2013). Mutualantagonism between the Ebola virus VP35 protein and the RIG-I activator pact determines infection outcome. Cell Host Microbe, 14:74–84.

[48] Edwards, M. R., Liu, G., Mire, C. E., Sureshchandra, S., Luthra, P., Yen, B., & Amarasinghe, G. K. (2016). Differential regulation of interferon responses by Ebola and Marburg virus VP35 Proteins. Cell Reports, 14(7):1632–1640.

[49] Madara, J. J., Han, Z., Ruthel, G., Freedman, B. D., & Harty, R. N. (2015). The multifunctional Ebola virus VP40 matrix protein is a promising therapeutic target. Future Virology, 10(5):537–546.

Chapter 7

Ebola Virus's Glycoproteins and Entry Mechanism

Khadija Khataby, Yassine Kasmi,
Rahma Ait Hammou, Fatima Ezzahra Laasri,
Said Boughribi and My Mustapha Ennaji

Additional information is available at the end of the chapter

http://dx.doi.org/10.5772/64032

Abstract

Ebola virus glycoprotein (GP) is the only protein that is expressed on the surface of the virus. The GP proteins play critical roles in the entry of virus into cell and in the evasion of the immune system. The GP gene transcript to membrane GP is constituted of two subunits GP1 and GP2,and the secretory GP (sGP). The main function of GP1/2 is to attach virus to target cell's membrane, whereas sGP has multiple functions on Ebola pathogenesis, such as inactivate neutrophils through CD16b causing lymphocyte apoptosis and vascular dysregulation. There are many studies that focused on better understanding the GP mechanism and aim at developing new antibodies and drugs such as VSV-EBOV, cAd3-EBO Z, rVSVN4CT1 VesiculoVax, 'C-peptide' based on the GP2 C-heptad repeat region (CHR) targeted to endosomes (Tat-Ebo) and MBX2270. In this chapter, we discuss the Ebola viral glycoproteins, genomic organization, synthesis, and their roles and functions. On the other hand, we treat the mechanisms of pathogenicity associated with Ebola GPs.

Keywords: EBOLA, virus, glycoprotein (GP), entry, mechanism, pathogenesis, structure

1. Introduction

Since the beginning of the year 2012, cases of Ebola virus have been reported in four African countries: Guinea, Liberia, Sierra Leone and Nigeria. WHO announced the end of Ebola outbreak in January 2016 [1]; despite this, according to the WHO, new cases are declared later in Sierra Leone, Liberia and Guinea [2, 3]. What this highlights is that the risk of the Ebola epidemic is still standing. The Ebola haemorrhagic fever weans and is often fatal in humans. It is caused by *Filoviridae*, citing the species Zaire Ebola virus (ZEBOV).

Ebola virus is a pathogenic agent of Ebola haemorrhagic fever; it is a single-stranded RNA with negative sense and with a genome length of approximately 18,920 nucleotides. Since it belongs to *Filoviridae*, its diameter is about 80 nm with a twisted filamentous form. Generally, the virus length is up to 1.1 μm [4], but particles of 14 μm were detected in the culture of liver tissue [5]. The viral RNA contains information about eight proteins, VP24, VP30, VP35, VP40, L, NP, sGP and GP1/2. Each of the protein expressed by EBOV is known for its multi-functionality that is why it is nominated as Swiss Army Knife, essentially VP35 and GP that present multi-functionality in the pathogenesis process and in the inhibition of immune responses in the host. EBOV is classified as a Category A priority pathogen by the National Institute of Allergy and Infectious Diseases (NIAID) and a Category A agent of bioterrorism by the Centers of Disease Control and Prevention (CDC) [6].

The principal characteristics of the Ebola virus is the presence of a heavily glycosylated GP on the external surface of viral membrane. Crystallographic studies revealed that GP on the viral surface exists in the trimeric form [7].

This chapter aims to provide a current overview on the treatment of GP of the Ebola virus, genomic organization, synthesis, their roles and functions, and the mechanisms of viral entry associated with GP and replication.

2. Phylogenetic information of Ebola virus

A total of 132 sequences are collected from the NCBI gene database. The samples were collected from the Makona river (80 sequences from Sierra Leon and 52 from Guinea), and they were collected in the period between 1 June 2014 and 30 August 2015. They underwent a global alignment and phylogenetic analysis by MEGA 6.4 and BEAST [8, 9].

Phylogenetic analysis reveals a greater genetic diversity with the presence of three distinct lines. The first line represents a set of sequences found only in Guinea, and that is most closely

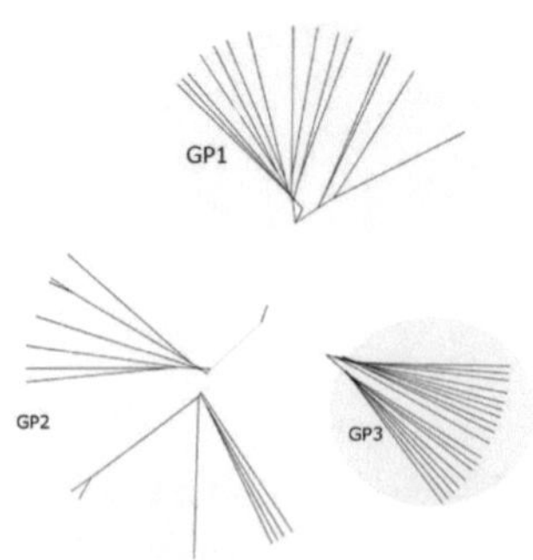

Figure 1. Phylogram of Ebola virus obtained with BEAST, the phylogenic software based on Bayesian evolutionary analysis. The first cluster (GP1) contains sequences from Guinea alone. In second cluster (GP2), we may find sequences from Sierra Leone and Guinea. In third cluster (GP3), the sequences from Fore'cariah, Dalaba are collected.

related to viruses taken early in March 2014. The cluster found in the large Conakry region is relative to two other lines. The second cluster contains sequences from Sierra Leone and Guinea; it could be a reintroduction of Sierra Leone or Guinea streaming in related strains to those initially introduced in Sierra Leone. Finally, a third group of viruses is located in Conakry, Fore'cariah, Dalaba, and to a limited extent in Coyah. Several sequences from Sierra Leone are grouped within the third cluster. Such phylogenetic structure suggests that there have been multiple migrations of EBOV into Guinea from Sierra Leone [10, 11]. However, following the phylodynamic studies, the virus had accumulated a significant number of mutations, 7×10^{-4} substitutions per site per year [12]. **Figure 1** represents a phylogram of the Ebola virus.

3. Structural roles and genomic information on gylcoprotein

The Ebola genome mainly consists of seven genes, which encode eight proteins. Genes are delimited by conserved transcriptional signals; each gene starts with an initiation site at 3′ and ends with a (polyadenylation) stopover site. Zaire Ebola virus (EBOV) is a member of *Filoviridae* order of *Mononegavirales*. According to the ICTV (International Committee on Taxonomy of Viruses) classification, *Mononegavirales* order contains four families in addition to *Filoviridae,* which are *Bornaviridae, Nyamiviridae, Paramyxoviridae* and *Rhabdoviridae.*

Families of the *Mononegavirales* can be distinguished by the size of the genome and coding capacity, virion's morphology (filamentous, pleomorphic, or ball-shaped and bacilliform), viral pathogenesis and by its hosting organism. The nomenclature *Filoviridae* was changed several times for various reasons and also due to the nature of information discovered through the study of these viruses. The aim was to prepare a classification that reflects the knowledge and correct the international code of nomenclature [13]. Unfortunately, in the *Filoviridae* case, approaching ICTV has not been useful because both species and virus names had already been implemented in non-Latinized binomial form [14, 15]. The new nomenclature writes "***Zaire ebolavirus***" means the species "**Ebola virus,**" which is a member of Zaire Ebola virus—and is the most common member. However, the abbreviation is "EBOV." The new classification also contains a new genre called "**Cuevavirus,**" which is newly discovered and contains the species "*Lloviu cuevavirus*" [14].

The common characteristics of this family are as follows: a negative genome RNA, which is linear, single-stranded, mono-segmented and filamentous; the genes in genome are ordered in specific ways, always starting with gene for envelope protein (3′UTR) and finishing with gene for the RNA polymerase (5′UTR); the viral replication occurs after synthesizing anti-genome; RNA is stored within the helical nucleocapsid; and RNA polymerase gene is the largest gene of *Filoviridae* [16].

Besides the common characteristics, there are others that allow the distinctions between the genomes of *Filoviruses* from *Mononegavirales* order, such as the location of overlapping genes in *Filoviridae.* Overlaps are of the length 18–20 bases and are limited to the conserved sequences determined for transcription signals [17]. The bioinformatics analysis of the amino acids' sequences of the protein from *Filoviridae* has shown different degrees of identities. The analysis has shown that the nucleoprotein (NP) is the most conserved protein with a significant identity with the exception of the C-terminal portion. The rates of conservation for other proteins are as follows: 33% for VP35, 27% for VP40, 34% for GP, 33% for VP30 and 37% for VP24 [17–19].

In **Figure 2**, the genome of EBOV is shown schematically. From this scheme it is evident that the fourth gene from the 3′ of the viral genome encodes for glycoprotein (GP). This gene contains two reading frames: GP is one of the genes that encode for two mRNA—ORF I of the GP gene encodes for an sGP of about 50–70 kDa (it is non-structural glycoprotein that is efficiently secreted by infected cells) and ORF II encodes for a transmembrane glycoprotein of 120–150 kDa. The length of this gene is about 2406 nucleotides and is located between nucleotide 5900 and 8308. It is located before the VP40 gene and after the VP30 gene.

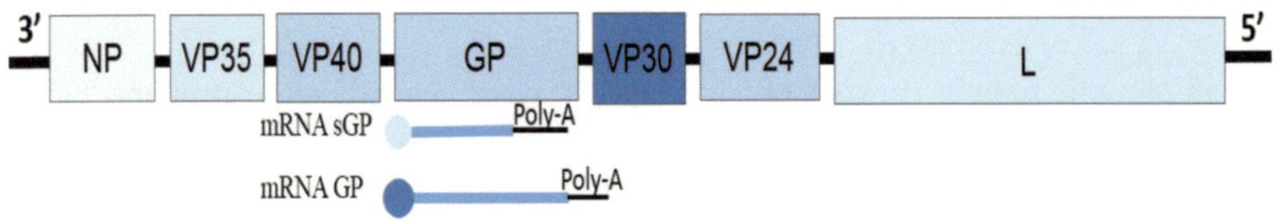

Figure 2. The full length genome of Ebola is about 19,000 base, where L is the length of the gene and is more conserved then the VP40, which is the more polymorphisized gene; however, the GP is within an average polymorphism. The sequence 6.039–6.923 coding for the GP1 is followed by polyadenine before the GP2 sequence in position 6.924–8.068.

The GP gene is localized between the nucleotides 5883 and 8288, where the mRNA of small non-structural secreted glycoprotein is encoded between the regions 6022 and 7116; however, the membrane GP is encoded by the regions 6022 and 8051 of nucleotides, where the region 6022–6906 is responsible for the subunit GP1 and the nucleotide sequence form 6906 to 8051 in the EBOV's genome coding is responsible for GP2; here we observed that for sGP and GP1/2 the coding starts separately.

The GP gene advances by conserved transcription start and stop signals: "CUACUUC UAAUU" as the start transcription signal for nucleotides 5883 and 5894, and "UAAUUCU" as the stop transcription signal. The end of the gene of GP containing a region encoding (UUUUUU) or including that of the GP gene (UAAUUCUUUUU) is typically sited in the region 8278–8288. It is plausible to think that the purpose of these poly U's into the genome, and these sites, is to form a poly-adenine during the transcription for retaining the mRNA and forming a premature protein [19].

A major difference between the Ebola and Marburg species has been shown with regards to the GP gene. In contrast to Ebola in which the genome contains information about two different forms of GP (sGP and GP), the GP gene of Marburg only codes a single GP.

The work of Sullivan et al. [20] has dismissed that a single mutation in the position 77 or 121 in the sequence of GP2 is able to influence the cytotoxicity and the immunogenicity of the virus. A post-transcriptional modification is also able to have the same effect [20]. The post-transcriptional change may be due to the effects of prophylactic drugs or antibodies that are specifically reactive with the GP2 [20]. The structure of EBOV GP and its interaction with the

http://dx.doi.org/10.5772/64032

human antibody KZ52 is shown in **Figure 3**. Therefore, the GP1 subunit of GP binds with the GP2 subunit by a non-covalent bond; therefore, the residues of GP at the positions 266 and 476 do not significantly affect viral entry [21].

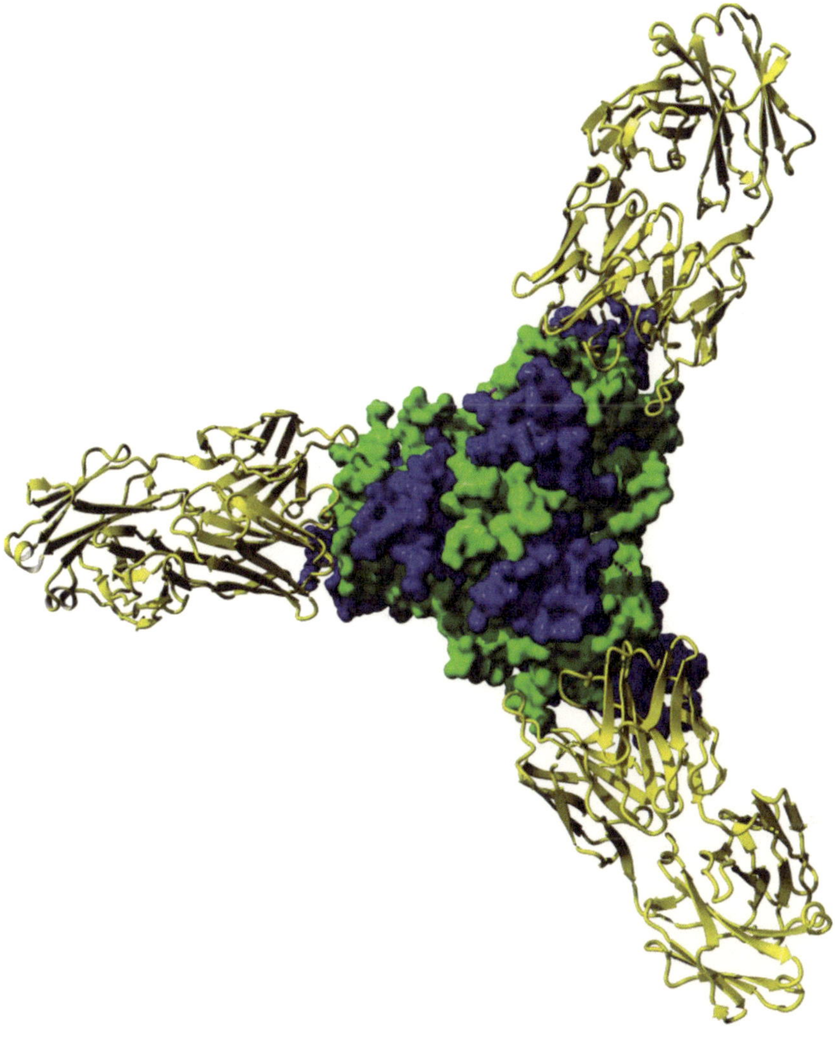

Figure 3. The Ebola virus glycoprotein has a calyx structure-like tribal as it is demonstrated by the crystal structure. According to the crystal structure of the protein, it is shown that three subunits of GP1 (blue) are bound to three GP2's subunits (green). In yellow it is shown that the human antibody KZ52 interacted with the GP at the base of the chalice [7, 14].

Multiple studies have shown that the GP gene products have the following multiple roles in the process of pathogenesis:

- The binding to the receptor is performed by the GP1 subunit whereas the GP2 subunit is responsible for the fusion and viral entry [22].

- Cytopathic effects: cell rounding and detachment.

- The EBOV secretory GP is incriminated in the provocation of B and T lymphoid apoptosis, but an investigation suggests that the soluble GP has no role in apoptosis [23]. It is also involved in antigenic subversion as well as restoring the barrier function of endothelial cells [6].

4. Synthesis of GP and maturation

4.1. The transmembrane glycoprotein GP1/2

EBOV GP has 676 amino acids in length with an apparent molecular weight of 150 kDa. The glycoprotein is synthesized as a precursor of pre-GP (or GP0) considering the length of the gene. A series of post-translational events leads to the maturation of the viral glycoprotein, *N*-glycosylation of the protein in the endoplasmic reticulum and the *O*-glycosylation in the Golgi. The pre-GP precursor is finally cleaved in the trans-Golgi compartment by a protease, furin, into two subunits: extracellular GP1(501 amino acids) and the GP2 transmembrane subunit (175 amino acids), which are interconnected together by disulphide bridges [24]. GP plays a role in the pathogenesis through regulation of the adaptive response. It is at the origin of [24]

- reduction with the availability of adhesion molecules;

- disruption of the presentation of the viral antigens to lymphocytes; and

- glycoproteins GP1 and GP2 have immunosuppressive motifs.

4.2. The secretory glycoprotein (sGP)

We hypothesize that the alteration of the homeostasis system and vascular system observed during Ebola virus disease could be, at least in part, caused by these soluble glycoproteins [25].

Recent works show that the source of the expression of GP1/2 or sGP is the ribosomal slippage process, where eight adenines nucleotides play an important role in the inversion of the expression of sGP and GP1/2,.If the transcription complex reads only seven adenines, it encodes for the secretory GP, while the reading of the eight adenines leads to the transcription of the pre-GP1/2 by dint of two disulphide-linked subunits GP1 and GP2. **Figure 4** illustrates this translational frameshifting or ribosomal frameshifting shown in the Ebola virus GP gene [26].

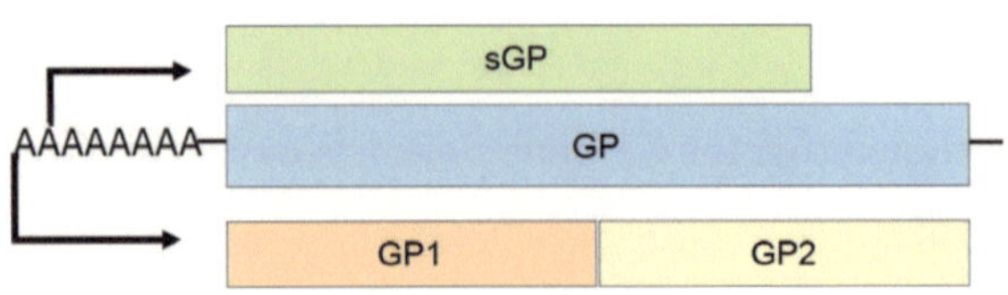

Figure 4. Illustration of the translational frameshifting of the GP gene due to the open reading frame.

5. Viral cycle and pathogenicity

The pathogenesis mechanism of the Ebola virus begins with the infection of the immune system's cells such as macrophages, dendritic cells (DCs) and monocytes, which are the first that come to contact with the viral particles. An alteration of interferon's production is observed in the infected cells, and the level of alteration is different from one cell to another. DCs and monocytes are the cells that show important level of alterations and, consequently, the INF production level decreases significantly. Furthermore, lymphocyte apoptosis and a global dysfunction of specific immune system's cells are observed with the increase of viral burden. In addition, the virus is responsible for other dysfunctions such as neutrophils inactivation, induction of apoptosis, inhibitor of immune response, and involvement in the process of viral entry in epithelial cells, vascular dysregulation and evasion [24, 27, 28]. The spread of virus throughout the body including the vital organs with immune system dysfunction leads to death.

The Ebola virus attacks the whole body causing increasing disseminated intravascular coagulation that degrades quickly the haemostasis and the functioning of vital organs. Infection destroys the endothelial cells, mononuclear phagocytes (monocytes, macrophages, dendritic cells, mast cells) and hepatocyte [29]. The mechanism of pathogenicity and the viral cycle can be divided into three phases:

- State extracellular and penetration, which cited the paramount role of the GP and GSP.

- State intracellular and the role of replication complex.

- Roles of VP24, VP40 and VP35 in the evasion of the immune system.

5.1. Target cells and receptors

The tropism of the Ebola virus depends on the expression of the receptor at the entry of the virus by the target cell. Several receptors of *Filoviridae* were determined.

The Ebola GP is bound to the C-type lectins as DC-SIGN, L-SIGN and hMGL expressed by monocytic, dendritic and macrophage cells [30–33]. The virus uses other ubiquitous molecules expressed by non-monocytic cells to internalize the target cells too [34]. The Ebola virus also uses a process called antibody-dependent enhancement (ADE) to attach the host cells and facilitate the entry [35]. It is shown that the GP binds with the IgG Fc receptor IIIb and forms a cross-linking virus-antibody-complement complex to Fcγ III, which explains the rapid spread of virus throughout the body (liver, brain, heath and endothelial cell) [35]; other study demonstrated that T-cell immunoglobulin and mucin domain 1 are receptors for the Ebola virus [35].

The Ebola virus infects most types of cells. However, macrophages and dendritic cells allow a strong replication and spread of the virus through the lymph and blood circulatory system. Thus, the virus reaches lymph nodes, liver and spleen, and spreads to other tissues.

5.2. Extracellular role of GP

The infective dose of EBOV is about 1–10 virion by aerosol in non-human primates. Despite this small amount of the virus, the formation and composition of the virion allows it to cause problems for the infected bodies.

However, after infection, it tries to prevent and interfere with the immune response via glycoproteins EBOV (GP), which is one of the reasons why the Ebola virus is fatal. The EBOV glycoprotein is the only viral protein expressed on the surface of the virion and is essential for binding to host cells and the catalysis of membrane fusion in addition to other roles of pathogenicity. The GP is combined with carbohydrates that help in the prevention of the immune system; also, the coating of the protein in a sweet layer makes it more difficult for the immune system to identify that a virus is present. On the other hand, the GP released into the intracellular medium inhibited host antibodies. It is also accompanied by the rapid neutralization of certain populations of T lymphocytes by a super-antigen effect. The GP is the essential protein in the mechanism of penetration. The GP-secreted/transmembrane GP inhibit the effect of neutralization of the natural antibodies (Ab), thanks to the carbohydrates combined with GP. The GP related to Ab easily gets attached on the cell membrane by C1q (thanks to the complement immune). This attachment facilitates and promotes deposition on host cell and this is followed by the penetration of the virus via the macropinosome pathway (this is the same capture solute of intercellular lipid lane) to the cell. Moreover, citing the possibility of using the protein G and calthrin, it indicates the role of the actin in the penetration of virus and suggests that the virus promotes, locates and retakes a large part of it action by interactions (**Figure 5**).

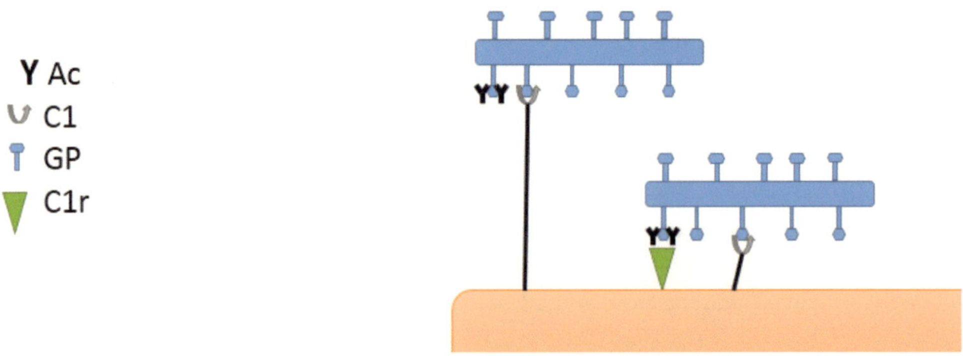

Figure 5. The mechanism of recognition and virus entry. GP binds to the antibodies of unknown site in the Fab regions. C1q complement allows the binding of the antibody bound to the virus with the target cells. The internalization of virus is the objective of multiple receptors known to the GP, they are of relatively non-specific type.

The GP binds with neutrophils and endothelial cells by the DC-SIGN (dendritic-cell-specific ICAM3-grabbing non-integrin) and L-SIGN (liver and lymph node SIGN), which provide links to cell-GP via carbohydrate determinants. These bonds formed with the neutrophil receptor CD16 cause a significant reduction in the signal CR3 and Fcγ receptor II B, avoiding virus clearance. It has been shown that the strong pro-inflammatory responses were induced by the commitment of the EBOV GP with the TLR-4 and by the activation of the NF-κB transcription factor. The GP is responsible for cytotoxicity on endothelial cells by secretion of enzymes, proteolytic endosomes (such as cathepsin), that cause the destruction of the vascular endo thelium and increase in vascular permeability and haemorrhagic signs.

In addition, the GP also binds with multiple nearby IgG, which allows the binding of C1 to the Fc region of antibodies that is thermo labile, and interacts with the cell surface molecules. This complex consists of C1q and two pro-enzymes of serine protease, C1r and C1s [26], which allow the virus to bind to cell membranes. At that time the virus enters and internalizes the cell via the macropinocytosis [36] (**Figure 6**).

The amount of BST2 into cell does not change but the surface of BST2 decreases in the presence of the GP. This explains that the GP hides the BST2 receptors in its absence, and VP40 that commune-precipitates and co-localizes binds with BST2. This reveals that GP plays a role in the inhibition of this interaction [37].

5.3. Intracellular action of GP

Macrophages and dendritic cells are the first to be infected, but the viruses can infect most cell types with the notable exception of lymphocytes and other non-adherent cells [38]. Several researches have shown that the EBOV's binding with the receptors is relatively non-specific. For example, EBOV may also attach to C-type lectins, which interact with glycans on EBOV GP as well as on phosphatidylserine (PtdSer) receptors which interacts with the viral envelope, which leads to a better EBOV entry [39, 40]. PtdSer receptors include Gas6 or protein S and TAM family receptors (TYRO3, AXL and MER).

It is suggested that EBOV enters cells through endocytosis clathrin [41]. The typical architecture of Ebola virions (length 1–2 μm, diameter 80–100 nm) is larger than the diameter of the clathrin-coated pits (85–110 nm).

It was found that their internalization was independent of clathrin- or caveolae-mediated endocytosis, but they co-localized with sorting nexin (SNX) 5 [42]. Once it is internalized, the virus must be carried in an intracellular compartment containing the factors essential for the activation of GP. The virus is initially inside the cell and in macropinosomes. The proteases cathepsin B and cathepsin L cysteine cleave GP and remove over 60% of the peptide mass, while interacting with NPC1 GP1 they intended to promote fusion of the viral membrane with the membrane of the bladder, accompanied with a pH drop in macropinosomes announcing the end of this step, which causes the fusion of the membrane of the host to the virus. Then, the complex transcription is released first, followed by the release of the viral genome [37, 43] (**Figure 6**).

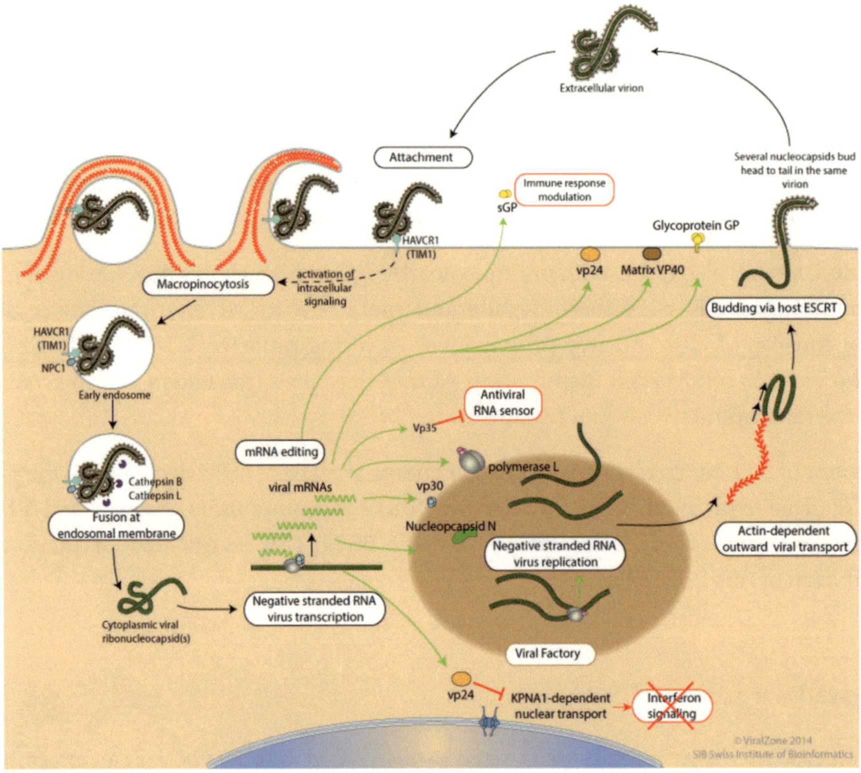

Figure 6. The diagram summarizes the virus entry mechanism and the various stages of internalization and replication. After attachment of the virus to the cell membrane, it activates the formation of macropinosomes via intracellular signals including the role of HAVCR1 (TM1), which recently has demonstrated the roles of the TIM-1 as a receptor or a cofactor for entry of Ebola virus. Moreover, the expression of endogenous TIM-1 reduced in very permissive cell lines leads to a reduction of the infectivity of Ebola virus [44]. Cleavage of the GP via Cathepsin B and L allows the fusion of endosomal membrane with virus causing the release of virus into the cytoplasm. By order, the VP30, VP35 and L are the first that are released into the cytoplasm and the viral genome negative sb RNA (Image from ViralZone2014 [45]).

Transcription and replication complex, VP35, N and L ensure the transfer of RNA– to RNA+ for transcription and translation of viral genome. The first step is the activation of the transcription complex by the fixation of zinc in the active site (70–90) of co-activator VP30. The VP30 binds with VP35, L and N to start the transcription and translation. The mRNAs are translated using host ribosomes. At this point, we can say that *filoviridae* are independent in their replication machinery and they need only a transcriptional signal (zinc and ribosomes) from the host cell.

The maturation of the GP track in the Golgi apparel, where the GP sequence is cleaved into GP 1 and GP2, is expressed on the surface of the cytoplasmic membrane and sGP.

The VP35, VP24 and VP40 play roles in the inhibition of immune responses by inhibition of the translation and signalization of antiviral genes by the succession of kinase-phosphorylation reactions.

PDB-ID	Studied system	Macromolecule content	Experimental data
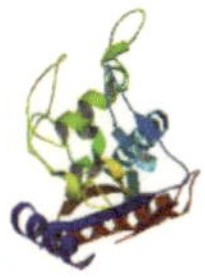 5F18	Structural basis of Ebola virus entry: viral glycoprotein bound to its endosomal receptor Niemann-Pick C1 Wang, H. (2016) Cell **164**: 258–268	Niemann-Pick C1	**Method:** X-ray diffraction **Resolution:** 2.00 Å **Residue Count:** 256 **DOI**: 10.2210/pdb5f18/pdb
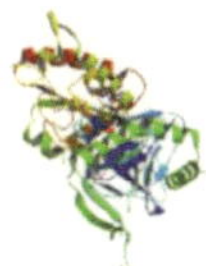 5F1B	Structural basis of Ebola virus entry: viral glycoprotein bound to its endosomal receptor Niemann-Pick C1 Wang, H. (2016) Cell **164**: 258–268	GP1, GP2, Niemann-Pick C1	**Method:** X-ray diffraction **Resolution:** 2.30 Å **Residue Count:** 544 **DOI**: 10.2210/pdb5f1b/pdb
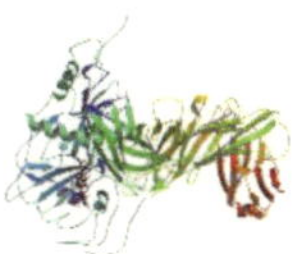 3VE0	Crystal structure of Sudan Ebolavirus Glycoprotein (strain Boniface) bound to 16F6 Bale, S., *et al.* (2012) Viruses **4**: 447–470	Envelope glycoprotein, 16F6 Antibody chain A,B	**Method:** X-ray diffraction **Resolution:** 3.35 Å **Residue Count:** 897 **DOI**: 10.2210/pdb3ve0/pdb
3CSY 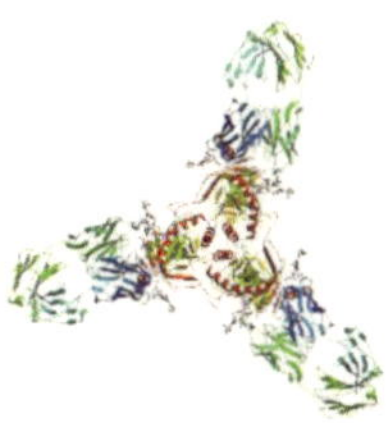	Crystal structure of the trimericprefusion Ebola virus glycoprotein in complex with a neutralizing antibody from a human survivor Lee, J.E., *et al.* (2008) Nature **454**: 177–182	Fab KZ52 heavy chain Fab KZ52 light chain Envelopeglycoprotein GP1 Envelopeglycoprotein GP2	**Method:** X-RAY DIFFRACTION **Resolution:** 3.40 Å **Residue Count:** 3632 **DOI**: 10.2210/pdb3csy/pdb
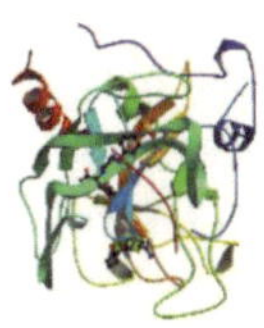 2QHR	Crystal structure of the 13F6-1-2 Fab fragment bound to its Ebola virus glycoprotein epitope. Lee, J.E. *et al.* (2008) J. Mol. Biol. **375**: 202–216	13F6-1-2 Fab fragment heavy chain 13F6-1-2 Fab fragment V lambda Envelope glycoprotein peptide	**Method:** X-RAY DIFFRACTION **Resolution:** 2.00 Å **Residue Count:** 451 **DOI**: 10.2210/pdb1qhr/pdb
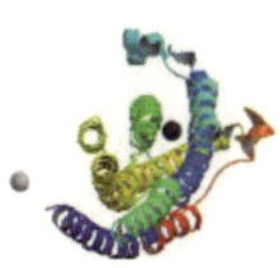 1EBO	Crystal structure of the Ebola virus membrane-fusion subunit, GP2, from the envenlope glycoprotein Weissenhorn, W. *et al.* (1998) Mol. Cell **2**: 605–616	Envelope glycoprotein GP2	**Method:** X-RAY DIFFRACTION **Resolution:** 3.00 Å **Residue Count:** 786 **DOI**: 10.2210/pdb1ebo/pdb
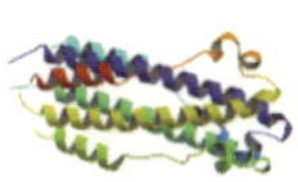 2EBO	Core structure of GP2 from Ebola virus Malashkevich, V.N. *et al.* (1999) Proc. Natl. Acad. Sci. USA **96**: 2662–2667	Envelope glycoprotein GP2	**Method:** X-RAY DIFFRACTION **Resolution:** 1.90 Å **Residue Count:** 222 **DOI**: 10.2210/pdb2ebo/pdb

Table 1. The collection of crystallographic structures related to Ebola's GP.

When the complex polymerase binds along the RNA template, the polymerase complex stops and is re-introduced at each junction of genes and transcription, thus individual genes appear sequentially in their 3′–5′ order. The region 3′ in the genome and anti-genome viral contains promoter's sites of replication for positive and negative sense RNA synthesis; they are approximately 176b [46]. The virus acts on microtubules and immunosuppressive genes to inhibit cell division. As the number of virions increases, it causes a burst of the host cell and then death or apoptosis due to the speed of the replication of virions, which are approximately 109 plaque-forming units (PFUs) in tissue during 7–10 days [26].

The spread of the virus in the body and vital organs causes haemorrhage and fever due to unskilled hyper activation of cytokines via transmembrane GP, and the activity of the NK causes diarrhoea because of the infection of digestive cells of the system. In addition, the pneumocystis, hepatocytes and cardiovascular cell infection accelerates the death of the patient.

5.4. Strategies for the inhibition of the *Ebola virus*

Several methods can be used to inhibit *filoviridae* and more particularly the glycoprotein. The inhibition of the GP induces entry cell inhibition and then limited viral infection. **Table 1** shows different crystalline forms of GP with cellular proteins, which develop the pathology and suggest a site to inhibit. Inhibitors must beagle to inhibit the alone active site of GP1 or both active sites of GP2. The inhibitors may be antibodies or small molecules that interact with EBOV proteins in the way to limit its action. The EBOV has the ability to use multiple ways as immune pathway, therefore it is important to design inhibitor or cocktail of inhibitors that inhibit multiple targets at the same time. In our opinion, the best way to reduce devastating action of EBOV is the collective inhibition of GP and VP30. The inhibition of GP is to reduce the side effects caused by the GP. Many antibodies and inhibitors were developed, and some of them during clinical trials [47]. However, the inhibition of VP30 is also the best way to inhibit the replication process and then remove the virus via mRNA degradation by RNAase.

6. Biosecurity, biosafety and Ebola virus

A good understanding of the mechanisms of the virus' action allows us to manipulate the viruses in the level of biosafety, which is lower than BSL-4. The virus is composed of two complementary and essential units for the infectious act, genome and VP30, VP35, VP40 and L proteins; merging of genome with these four proteins is capable of inducing infection. As Ebola is a negative sense single-stranded RNA virus, the isolation of their genome from its microenvironment composed of four proteins cannot trigger a viral reaction. As such Ebola cannot synthesize DNA genome, therefore, its cDNA copy is synthesized only in a laboratory, in which all manipulation conditions are easily manageable.

The best way to master and control the transcription and translation processes in the laboratory is by not allowing a transcription/translation of the total genome. Moreover, by isolating the proteins from their genome and other proteins, the pathogenic effects can be stopped. The pathogenic effect is caused by the cooperation and integration of different proteins that make up the genome of the viruses; however, the loss of a single protein causes the inhibition of virus by losing their genetic information via the degradation of cellular RNA as in the case of VP30.

It is possible to clone cDNA in *E. coli* in the BSL-2 laboratory [52, 53], which is consistent with the approach outlined in the BMBL and is responsible for developing and implementing an appropriate biosecurity measure. By cloning the cDNA of a gene, it is possible that it will accelerate the scientific research process and help in discovering new drugs. The study of individually cloned altered proteins is also possible in animals' models.

7. Conclusions

Based on the data presented in this chapter, Ebola has developed multiple pathways and modes for the evasion of the immune system and internalization in target cells. Further studies are necessary for a good understanding of the entry mechanism. However, the specific proteins of virus or even the cDNA genome disassociated of proteins can be studied in BSL-2 because the effects of virus depends on the presence of genome associated with structural and functional proteins, which allows to study the virus in laboratories at biosafety level 3 or 2. They may even accelerate the process of finding new inhibitors by pharmaceutical and vaccination companies.

Acknowledgements

The authors thank the Ministry of Higher Education, University Hassan II of Casablanca, Faculty of Sciences and Technics and the Laboratory of Virology, Microbiology, Quality and Biotechnologies/Ecotoxicology & Biodiversity-Team of Virology, oncology and medical Biotechnologies.

Author details

Khadija Khataby, Yassine Kasmi, Rahma Ait Hammou, Fatima Ezzahra Laasri,
Said Boughribi and My Mustapha Ennaji*

*Address all correspondence to: m.ennaji@yahoo.fr

Laboratory of Virology, Microbiology, Quality and Biotechnologies/Ecotoxicology & Biodiversity, Faculty of Sciences and Techniques, University Hassan II of Casablanca, Casablanca, Morocco

Khadija Khataby and Yassine Kasmi contributed equally to this work.

References

[1] http://www.who.int/mediacentre/news/releases/2016/ebola-zero-liberia/en/consult-ed, 20 April 2016.

[2] http://apps.who.int/ebola/current-situation/ebola-situation-report-30-march-2016

[3] http://who.int/mediacentre/news/statements/2016/liberia-ebola/en/

[4] Gatherer, D. The 2014 Ebola virus disease outbreak in West Africa, published online ahead of print May 2, 2014. DOI: 10.1099/vir.0.067199-0, J Gen Virol May 2014 Vir. 0.067199-0, Received 22 April 2014. Accepted 28 April 2014.

[5] Geisbert, T. W., & Jahrling, P. B. (1995). Differentiation of Filoviruses by electron microscopy. Virus Research 39(2–3): 129–150. PMID 8837880.

[6] De la Vega, M. A., Wong, G., Kobinger, G. P., & Qiu, X. (2015). The multiple roles of SGP in Ebola pathogenesis. Viral Immunology, 28(1): 3–9.

[7] Lee, J. E., Fusco, M. L., Hessell, A. J., Oswald, W. B., Burton, D. R., & Saphire, E. O. (2008). Structure of the Ebola virus glycoprotein bound to an antibody from a human survivor. Nature, 454(7201): 177–182.

[8] Drummond, A. J., Suchard, M. A., Xie, D., & Rambaut, .A (2012). Bayesian phylogenetics with BEAUti and the BEAST 1.7. Molecular Biology and Evolution 29: 1969–1973. Full text.

[9] Tamura, K., Dudley, J., Nei, M., & Kumar, S. (2007). MEGA4: Molecular Evolutionary Genetics Analysis (MEGA) software version 4.0. Molecular Biology and Evolution 24: 1596–1599. (Publication PDF at http://www.kumarlab.net/publications).

[10] Baize, S., Pannetier, D., Oestereich, L., Rieger, T., Koivogui, L., Magassouba, N. F., … & Tiffany, A. (2014). Emergence of Zaire Ebola virus disease in Guinea. *New England Journal of Medicine*, 371(15), 1418-1425.

[11] Dudas G, Rambaut A (2014) A phylogenetic analysis of Guinea 2014 EBOV Ebolavirus outbreak. PLoS Curr 6: 1229–123

[12] Carroll, S. A., et al. (2013). Molecular evolution of viruses of the family Filoviridae based on 97 whole-genome sequences. Journal of Virology. 87: 2608–2616. DOI:10.1128/JVI. 03118-12

[13] King, A. M. Q., Adams, M. J., Carstens, E. B., & Lefkowitz, E. J. (2011). The international code of virus classification and nomenclature. In: King, A. M. Q., Adams, M. J., Carstens, E. B., & Lefko-Witz, E. J. (editors). Virus taxonomy—Ninth Report of the International Committee on Taxonomy of Viruses. Elsevier/Academic Press, London, pp. 1273–1277.

[14] Kuhn, J. H., Becker, S., Ebihara, H., Geisbert, T. W., Johnson, K. M., Kawaoka, Y., Lipkin, W. I., Negredo, A. I., Netesov, S. V., Nichol, S. T., Palacios, G., Peters, C. J., Ten-Orio, A., Volchkov, V. E., Jahrling, P. B. (2010). Proposal for a revised taxonomy of the family

filoviridae: classification, names of taxa and viruses, and virus abbreviations. Archives of Virology 155 (12): 2083–2103. DOI: 10.1007/S00705-010-0814-X. PMC 3074192. PMID 21046175

[15] Bukreyev, A. A., Chandran, K., Dolnik, O., Dye, J. M., Ebihara, H., Leroy, E. M.,... & Kuhn, J. H. (2014). Discussions and decisions of the 2012–2014 International Committee on Taxonomy of Viruses (ICTV) Filoviridae Study Group, January 2012–June 2013. Archives of Virology, 159(4): 821–830.

[16] Pringle, C. R. (1997). The order mononegavirales-current status. Archives of Virology 142.11: 2321–2326.

[17] Bukreyev, A. A., Belanov, E. F., Blinov, V. M., & Netesov, S. V. (1995). Complete nucleotide sequences of Marburg virus genes 5 and 6 encoding vp30 and vp24 proteins. Biochemistry and Molecular Biology International 35: 605–613.

[18] Sanchez, A., Kiley, M. P., Klenk, H. D., & Feldmann, H. (1992). Sequence analysis of the mar-burg virus nucleoprotein gene: comparison to Ebola virus and other non-segmented negative-strand RNA viruses. Journal of General Virology 73: 347–357.

[19] Volchkova, V. A., Vorac, J., Repiquet-paire, L., Lawrence, P., & Volchkov, V. E. (2015). Ebola virus GP gene polyadenylation versus RNA editing. Journal of Infectious Diseases, JIV150.

[20] Sullivan, N., Chakrabarti, B., Yang, Z. Y., Pau, M. G., Goudsmit, J., & Nabel, G. (2015). U.S. Patent No. 9,012,618. Washington, DC: U.S. Patent and Trademark Office.

[21] Manicassamy, B., Wang, J., Jiang, H., & Rong, L. (2005). Comprehensive analysis of Ebola virus GP1 in viral entry. Journal of Virology, 79(8): 4793–4805.

[22] Takada, A., Robison, C., Goto, H., Sanchez, A., Murti, K. G., Whitt, M. A., & Kawaoka, Y. (1997). A system for functional analysis of Ebola virus glycoprotein. Proceedings of the National Academy of Sciences USA 94: 14764–14769.

[23] Russier, M. (2013). Cellules NK et fievres hemorragiques virales: etude de leur role dans la mise en place des reponses immunes et dans la pathogenese lors de l'infec-tion par les virus lassa et ebola. Doctoral Dissertation, ecole normale superieure de lyon-ens Lyon.

[24] Escudero-perez, B., Volchkova, V. A., Dolnik, O., Lawrence, P., & Volchkov, V. E. (2014). Shed GP of Ebola virus triggers immune activation and increased vascular permeability. PLOS Pathogens 10(11): e1004509.

[25] Mohan, G. S., Li, W., Ye, L., Compans, R. W., & Yang, C. (2012). Antigenic subversion: a novel mechanism of host immune evasion by Ebola virus. PLoS Pathogens 8(12): e1003065.

[26] Mohamadzadeh, M., Chen, L., & Schmaljohn, A. L. (2007). How Ebola and Mar-burg viruses battle the immune system. Nature Reviews Immunology 7(7): 556–567.

[27] Mohamadzadeh, M., Coberley, S. S., Olinger, G. G., Kalina, W. V., Ruthel, G., Fuller, C. L.,... & Schmaljohn, A. L. (2006). Activation of triggering receptor ex-pressed on myeloid cells-1 on human neutrophils by Marburg and Ebola viruses. Journal of Virology 80(14): 7235–7244.

[28] Geisbert, T. W., Young, H. A., Jahrling, P. B., Davis, K. J., Kagan, E., & Hensley, L. E. (2003). Mecha-nisms underlying coagulation abnormalities in Ebola hemorrhagic fever: overexpression of tissue factor in primate mono-cytes/macrophages is a key event. Journal of Infectious Diseases 188(11): 1618–1629.

[29] Garcia-vallejo, J. J., & Van Kooyk, Y. (2015). DC-sign. C-type lectin with prominent role in immune system. In Glycoscience: Biology and Medicine (pp. 649–659). Springer, Japan.

[30] Gillespie, L., Roosendahl, P., Ng, W. C., Brooks, A. G., Reading, P. C., & Londrigan, S. L. (2016). Endocytic function is critical for influenza a virus infection via DC-sign and l-sign. Scientific Reports, 6: 19428.

[31] Wang, H., Shi, Y., Song, J., Qi, J., Lu, G., Yan, J., & Gao, G. f. (2016). Ebola viral glycoprotein bound to its endosomal receptor Niemann-Pick C1. Cell 164(1): 258–268.

[32] Takada, A., Fujioka, K., Tsuiji, M., Morikawa, A., Higashi, N., Ebihara, H.,... & Kawaoka, Y. (2004). Human macrophage c-type lectin specific for galactose and n-acetylgalactosamine promotes filo-virus entry. Journal of Virology 78(6): 2943–2947.

[33] Zampieri, C. A., Sullivan, N. J., & Nabel, G. J. (2007). Immunopathology of highly virulent pathogens: insights from Ebola virus. Nature Immunology 8(11): 1159–1164.

[34] Brudner, M., Karpel, M., Lear, C., Chen, L., Yantosca, L. M., Scully, C.,... & Mungall, B. A. (2013). Lectin-dependent enhancement of Ebola virus infection via soluble and transmembrane c-type lectin receptors. PLoS One 8(4), e60838.

[35] Sui, J., & Marasco, W. A. (2002). Evidence against Ebola virus SGP binding to human neutrophils by a specific receptor. Virology 303(1): 9–14.

[36] Kondratowicz, A. S., Lennemann, N. J., Sinn, P. L., Davey, R. A., Hunt, C. L., et al. (2011). T-cell immunoglobulin and mucin domain 1 (TIM-1) is a receptor for Zaire Ebola virus and lake Victoria Marburgvirus. Proceedings of the National Academy of Sciences U S A. doi: 10.1073/pnas.1019030108

[37] Takada, A., Feldmann, H., Ksiazek, T., & Kawaoka, Y. (2003). Antibody-dependent enhancement of Ebola virus infection. Journal of Virology, 77(13): 7539–7544.

[38] Gustin, J. K., Bai, Y., Moses, A. V., & Douglas, J. L. (2015). Ebola virus glycoprotein promotes enhanced viral egress by preventing Ebola vp40 from associating with the host restriction factor bst2/tetherin. Journal of Infectious Diseases, JIV125.

[39] Dube, D., et al. (2010). Cell adhesion-dependent membrane trafficking of a binding partner for the Ebola virus glycoprotein is a determinant of viral entry. Proceedings of the National Academy of Sciences USA 107: 16637–16642.

[40] Moller-tank, S., & Maury, W. (2014). Phosphatidylserine receptors: enhancers of enveloped virus entry and infection. Virology 468–470c: 565–580.

[41] Mollertank, S., & Maury, W. (2015). Ebola virus entry: a curious and complex series of events. PLOS Pathogens, 11(4): e1004731.

[42] Nanbo, A., Imai, M., Watanabe, S., Noda, T., Takahashi, K., Neumann, G.,...& Kawaoka, Y. (2010). Ebolavirusis internalized into host cells via macropinocytosis in a viral glycoprotein-dependent manner. PLoS Pathogens 6(9): e1001121.

[43] White, J. M., & Schornberg, K. L. (2012). A new player in the puzzle of filovirus en-try. Nature Reviews Microbiology 10(5): 317–322.

[44] Kondratowicz, A. S., Lennemann, N. J., Sinn, P. l., Davey, R. A., Hunt, C. L., Mollertank, S., Meyerholz, D. K., Rennert, P., Mullins, R. F., Brindley, M., Sandersfeld, L. M., Quinn, K., Weller, M., Mccray, P. B., Chiorini, J., & Maury, W. (May 2011). "T-cell immunoglobulin and mucin domain 1 (TIM-1) is a receptor for Zaire Ebola virus and lake victoria marburgvirus". Proceedings of the National Academy of Sciences U.S.A. 108(20): 8426–8431. doi:10.1073/pnas.1019030108. pmc 3100998. pmid 21536871.

[45] http://viralzone.expasy.org/all_by_species/5016.html, consulted 4th April 2016.

[46] Mühlberger, E. 2007. Filovirus replication and transcription. Future Virol. 2:205–215

[47] Higgins, C. D., Koellhoffer, J. F., Chandran, K., & Lai, J. R. (2013). C-peptide inhibitors of Ebola virus glycoprotein-mediated cell entry: effects of conjugation to cholesterol and side chain–side chain crosslinking. Bioorganic & Medicinal Chemistry Letters 23(19): 5356–5360.

[48] Bukreyev, A., Volchkov, V. E., Blinov, V. M., & Netesov, S. V. (1993). The GP-protein of Marburg virus contains the region similar to the 'immunosuppressive domain' of oncogenic retrovirus p15 e proteins. FEBS Lettters 323: 183–187.

[49] Empig, C. J., & Goldsmith, M. A. (2002). Association of the caveola vesicular system with cellular entry by Filoviruses. Journal of Virology 76: 5266–5270.

[50] Wolf, K., Beimforde, N., Falzarano, D., Feldmann, H., & Schnittler, H. J. (2011). The Ebola virus soluble glycoprotein (sGP) does not affect lymphocyte apoptosis and adhesion to activated endothelium. Journal of Infectious Diseases 204(Suppl 3): S947–S952.

[51] Ravikiran, T., & Prasad, Y. (2014). Ebola virus disease: epidemic broke out in lateral Africa. Indo American Journal of Pharmaceutical Research 4(12): 5909–5918.

[52] Heinz Feldmann, "Ebola virus cDNA and the NIH guidelines for Ebola virus cDNA and the NIH guidelines for research involving recombinant DNA molecules research

involving recombinant DNA molecules", National Institutes of Health (NIH) Recombinant DNA Advisory Committee (RAC) 116th Meeting Tuesday, March 3–4, 2009

[53] Michael Buchmeier, "Ebola cDNA: Biosafety Risks and Biosecurity Concerns", National Institutes of Health (NIH) Recombinant DNA Advisory Committee (RAC) 116th Meeting Tuesday, March 3–4, 2009

Chapter 8

Strategies for the Development of Small Molecule Inhibitors of Ebola Viral Infection

Sebastian Pleško and Črtomir Podlipnik

Additional information is available at the end of the chapter

http://dx.doi.org/10.5772/63502

Abstract

The recent outbreak of Ebola viral disease (EVD) in West Africa reminded us that an effective anti-viral treatment still does not exist, despite the significant progress that has recently been made in understanding biology and pathology of this lethal disease. Currently, there are no approved vaccine and/or prophylactic medication for the treatment of EVD in the market. However, the serious pandemic potential of EVD mobilized research teams in the academy and the pharmaceutical industry in the effort to find an Ebola cure as fast as possible. In this chapter, we are giving the condensed review of different approaches and strategies in search of a drug against Ebola. We have been focusing on the review of the targets that could be used for *in silico, in vitro*, and/or *in vivo* drug design of compounds that interact with the targets in different phases of the Ebola virus life cycle.

Keywords: small molecule inhibitors, Ebola virus, drug design, protein targets, structure and action

1. Introduction

Ebola virus (EBOV) is a (-)ssRNA filovirus, known for its extreme insidiousness. Case fatality rates of the current 2014 outbreak in West Africa are 50–70% [1]. Transmission of EBOV is predominantly via physical contact with bodily fluids of infected people or corpses and can be limited by a proper combination of early diagnosis, contact tracing, isolation of patients, infection control, and safe burial [2, 3].

The infection is characterized by suppression of the immune system and of the systemic inflammatory response, followed by the collapse of the vascular and immune systems, and multi-organ failure. The patient dies from a combination of dehydration, massive bleeding, and shock. Currently, there are no approved drugs for the hemorrhagic fever caused by EBOV. However, there is some conflicting clinical evidence that antibodies isolated from survived patients may be effective in the treatment of the infection caused by EBOV [4, 5].

In this book chapter, we will review possible targets that are being used or could be used for structure-based design of small molecule inhibitors against EBOV. We will start the chapter with a brief review of the structure and action of EBOV, and then we will describe the targets along with possible hotspots. Additionally, we will present a short review of small molecules that could be used as medicaments against EBOV.

2. Structure and action of Ebola virus

Knowledge about the life cycle of EBOV, supported with structural information, is crucial for the successful design of antivirals. This is the reason why we will start our review with the structural information about EBOV.

The RNA genome of Ebola virus contains information for constructing seven proteins (GP, VP24, VP30, VP35, VP40, L-protein, nucleoprotein), which assemble with the genomic RNA to form one of the most lethal viruses [6]. EBOV's RNA exists in antisense form, which means that it cannot be used for proteins' production directly [7]. For protein building, the complementary copy of the negative RNA is required, which is produced with the help of the viral polymerase (L-protein). Not all genes are transcribed fully through. For example, transcription of GP gene could lead to three different proteins: GP, sGP, and ssGP. A small nonstructural sGP (secretory glycoprotein) is the protein that is efficiently secreted from infected cells. sGP acts as mimic of full GP that is presented at the surface of EBOV, this mimicry is one of the ways of how the Ebola virus deceive the immune system, by urging the body to develop antibodies to sGP instead of full GP [8, 9]. EBOV is enclosed by a membrane hijacked from an infected cell and covered with Ebola glycoproteins. A layer of matrix proteins supports the membrane on the inside and holds a cylindrical nucleocapsid at the center, which stores and delivers the RNA genome.

The main task of Ebola glycoprotein (GP) is binding to receptors located on a host-cell surface and getting the Ebola genome inside. GP is distributed throughout the whole viral membrane surface and the large proportion of oligosaccharides, which are attached to the GP making the virus unrecognizable for the adaptive immune system. GP is a highly dynamic protein that snaps into different shapes when it binds to a cell surface, driving the virus close enough to get fused with the membrane.

The viral matrix is composed of two proteins: VP40 and VP24. The function of VP40, known as the major matrix protein, is to assist in the process of budding. VP40 hexamers form layers that support the nucleocapsid in the middle of the virion. The minor matrix protein VP24 is involved in interferon antagonism.

Another important structural element of EBOV is the nucleocapsid, which is located in the middle of the virion. The nucleocapsid is wound in a regular helix shape 50 nm in diameter. The nucleocapsid is composed of a series of viral proteins, which are attached to EBOV's genome, 19 kb linear, negative-sense RNA. The nucleocapsid is composed from the inner part where RNA is packed with NP protein, and the outer shell is composed of VP24, VP30, VP35, and polymerase (L-protein).

The detailed cross section through EBOV illustrated by Goodsell is shown in **Figure 1** [10].

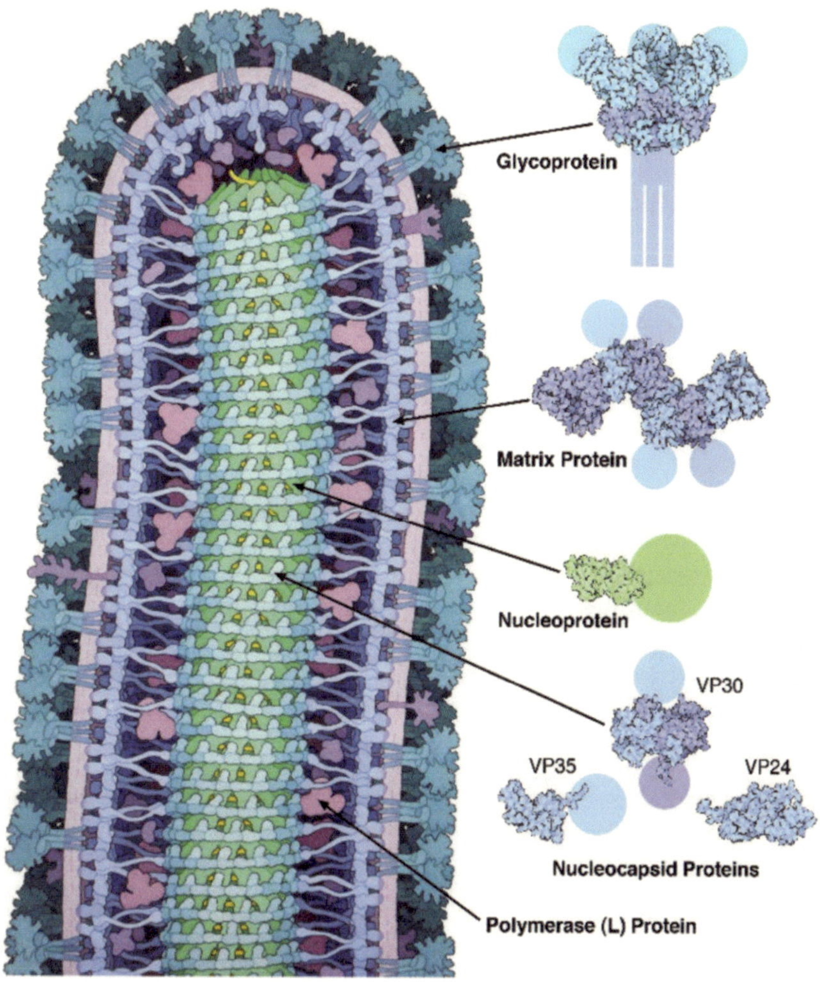

Figure 1. Cross section through of EBOV virion. The proteins are shown in blue, green, and magenta, the RNA genome in yellow, and the membrane in purple. The detailed structures are shown to the right. The nonresolved portions are shown with schematic circles (doi: 10.2210/rcsb_pdb/mom_2014_10).

The information about the function of EBOV's proteins about its structural data along with potential targets is collected in **Table 1**.

Protein	Function	Structures	Potential target for the protein
NP	Nucleocapsid and inclusion of body formation; encapsulation of RNA genome, replication and transcription of viral genome. Binds VP35, and associates with VP30 and L.	PDB structures: 4z9p, 4ypi, 4zta	target interactions with or binding sites on VP35, VP30 and L
VP35	Associates in RNP complexes, binds RNA. Together with L, it forms replicase–trancriptase holoenzyme, initiates transcription. EBOV VP35 suppresses Type-I IFN production.	PDB structures: 4qaz,4qb0,4ypi, 4z9p,4zta,4ztg, 4zti	Target basic patch of VP35 around the Arg312 to prevent VP35 binding to double stranded DNA (dsRNA) and promote IFN production.
VP40	Viral matrix protein. Accumulates at cellular membrane proliferation sites, responsible for viral budding. Associtesa with microtubules and outer cell membranes.	PDB structures: 1h2c, 1h2d, 2kq0, 4eje, 4ldb, 4ldd, 4ldi, 4ldm	Compound 5539-0062 inhibits interaction of VP40 with Tsg101 a factor involved in endosomal protein sorting.
GP1,2	Transmembrane protein that mediates viral attachment to the cell membrane and promote viral entry. Some domains of this protein may have immunosuppressive properties.	PDB structures: 2ebo, 2rlj, 3csy, 5f18,5f1b	Disruption of interaction between primed EBOV-GP and NPC1. Interaction of EBOV-GP with neutralizing antibodies (ZMAPP).
VP30	Secondary nucleoprotein, binds NP and ssRNA, part of ribonucleoprote-in complex. VP30 in oligomeric form is neded for the activation of transcription.	PDB structures: 2i8b, 3v7o, 5dvw	Target basic patch around LYS 180 to inhibit the activation of transcription.
VP24	Secondary matrix protein, it colocalizes with VP40 and has important function in nucleocapsid formation. VP24 inhibits cellular responses to IFN.	PDB structures: 3vne, 3vnf, 4d9o, 4m0q, 4or8, 4u2x	Inhibition of VP24 binding to karyopherin.
L protein	RNA dependent RNA polymerase; binds VP35 to form replicase transcriptional factor.	Only sequence	Poly-adenylation, profreading function or interaction with ZAP

This is based on a template by Shurtleff *et al.* [11].

Table 1. EBOV protein functions and availability of structural information[a].

3. Collection of targets for small molecule inhibitor design

In this section, we describe different targets and strategies for structure-based design of EBOV's small molecule inhibitors. Based on the knowledge of EBOV action, different strategies for curing Ebola viral disease are proposed: prevention of EBOV adhesion to host cells (monoclonal antibodies; inhibitors of host-cell receptors, ...) [12]; inhibition of viral escape from endosome (inhibition of NPC1, protease inhibitors) [13]; reviving and enhancing intracellular innate immunity; orthogonal RNA destruction mechanism targeting essential Ebola genes; inhibiting viral RNA processing (inhibition of RNA polymerase) [14]; disruption of viral assembly (nucleoprotein, VP40, VP24, VP35), etc.

Some of these mechanisms will be described in this section along with proposed targets. The ideogram where the connection between Ebola virus life cycle and possible therapeutic targets is shown in **Figure 2**.

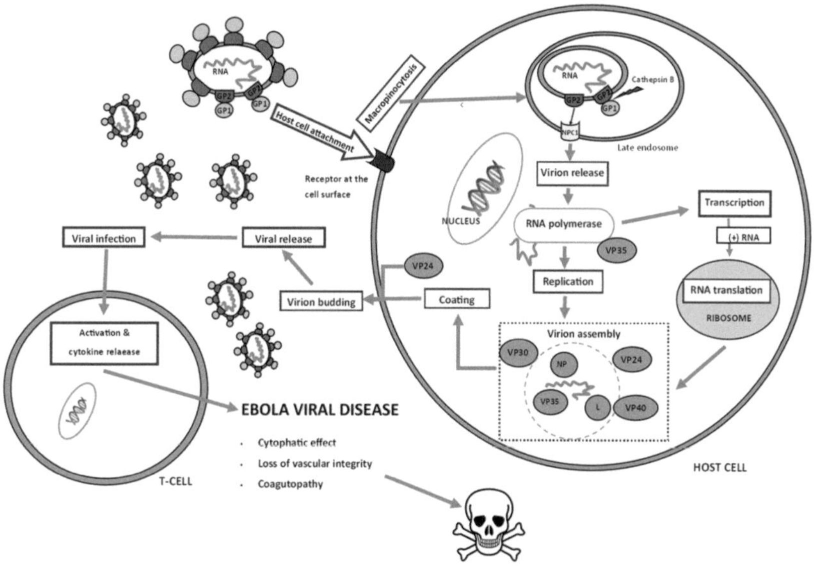

Figure 2. The ideogram of EBOV life cycle along with connections between possible therapeutic targets for the treatment EVD.

3.1. Nucleoprotein

The main function of nucleoprotein (NP) is encapsulation of the viral genome. EBOV's RNA located in the cage assembled mainly from nucleoprotein, which serves also as a scaffold for additional viral proteins forming nucleocapsid, is protected from the action of nucleases. The model of cross-section of RNA's cage composed from NP and VP35, based on recent X-ray diffraction structure (PDB-ID:4ypi) is shown in **Figure 3** [15]. A possible strategy to fight against EBOV is to prevent assembly of the RNA's cage. Binning *et al.* showed an elegant way to disrupt interaction between VP35 and nucleoprotein that is important for viral nucleocapsid's formation, by binding RNA aptamers [16]. Using electron microscopy technique, Noda *et al.* clearly showed that coexistence of NP and VP35 in proper ratio is important for nucleocapsid assembly [17]. Recently, Kirchdoerfer *et al.* have established that the N-terminal portion of VP35 acts as a chaperone for the viral nucleoprotein NP. They have also shown that VP35 prevents premature RNA binding and oligomerization of NP. Removal of VP35 peptide leads to NP self-assembly, which likely causes a conformational change between NP N- and C-terminal domains, facilitating RNA binding. The detailed knowledge of interactions between NP and VP35, supported with structural information (PDB-IDs: 4zta, 4zti, and 4ztg), which are conserved among filoviruses could provide key targets for structure-based drug design [18].

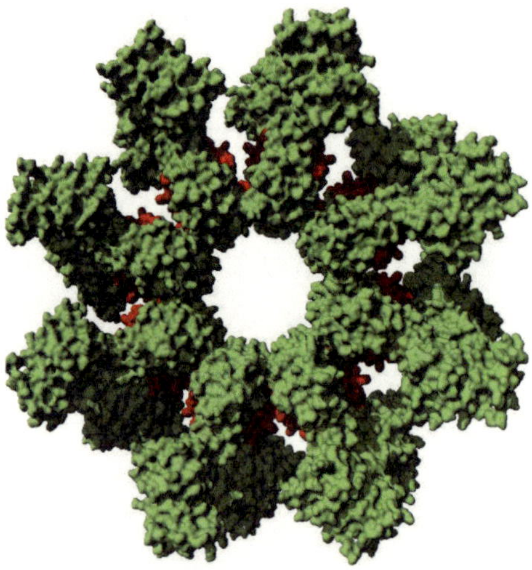

Figure 3. A model of axial cross section of the inner part of EBOV's RNA cage assembled from nucleoprotein (green) and VP35 (red). A model is based on PDB-ID:4ypi. YASARA (http://www.yasara.org) was used for visualization.

3.2. VP35 as a target for EVD therapeutics

EBOV's VP35 protein is a multifunctional protein, together with nucleoprotein and RNA, which is the main building block for the assembly of the nucleocapsid. Another important function of this protein is inhibition of interferon IFN-α/β production [19]. Additionally, VP35 is also a cofactor of the viral RNA polymerase. In this subsection, we will introduce the strategy for inhibition of VP35's polymerase activity with small molecules.

Using well-established *in silico* methods, followed by biological tests, NMR validation, and X-ray ligand:receptor structures, Brown *et al.* identified pyrrolidinone-based structures as promising inhibitors [20]. The ability of the identified compounds to inhibit interactions between VP35 and NP was evidently confirmed *in vitro* and by cell-based assay. The structure of inhibitor GA107 within the binding pocket of VP35 is shown in **Figure 4**. From the interaction map (**Figure 4A**), we may observe numerous contacts between GA107 and VP35's hydrophobic residues, including highly conserved Val 245, Ile 295, and Phe 328. This binding mode is also supported by two hydrogen bonds with Lys 251 and Gln 241. The authors of presented study have also shown that removal of either carboxylic acid or ketone moieties rapidly eliminates binding of certain ligands to the receptor. This fact is interesting from the aspect that Lys 251 is important for the VP35 polymerase cofactor function, as mutations at Lys 251 lead to loss of

http://dx.doi.org/10.5772/63502

this function [21]. Detailed molecular dynamics study of interaction of complexes between inhibitors and VP35 have revealed induced structural changes of the VP35 protein during binding event [22].

Inspired by the success of Brown *et al.*, we used Glide XP docking program to check the possibility of binding some small molecules, from our small in-house library of polyphenolic compounds [23], to the VP35 target. Surprisingly, we found that EGCG-green tea polyphenol could also nicely fit a druggable pocket of the protein. The pose of EGCG within VP35 IID is shown in **Figure 4B**. The number of hydrogen bonding contacts is greater than in the case of GA107 binding. The interaction between EGCG and VP35's Lys 251 is not detected in this case, but it is possible due to plasticity of the receptor site.

Ebola virus specifically inhibits the dsRNA (double stranded RNA) within cells via a sequestration process. The molecular basis of such sequestration is shown in **Figure 5**, where the complex between VP35 and model of dsRNA is presented. Mutagenesis studies have shown that critical residues for binding dsRNA are Phe 239, Arg 312, Arg 322, and Lys 339. Mutation of these residues to Ala results in VP35 complete loss of its ability to bind dsRNA, and thus were also unable to suppress IFN-β promoter [24]. Compounds like Ampligen, a immunomodulatory double stranded RNA, may be able to overcome this deficiency in host response [24, 25].

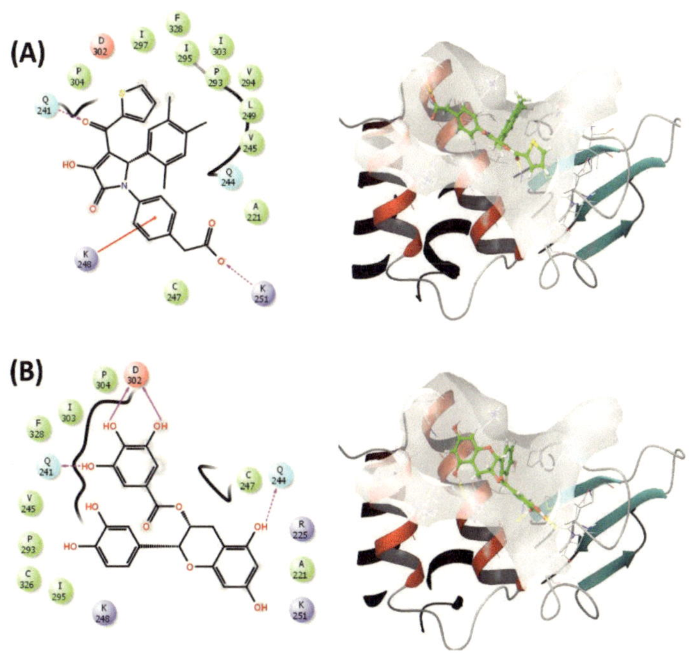

Figure 4. The interaction of compound GA017 (A) and EGCG (B) with proposed binding site of VP35. A docking protocol using Schrodinger's Glide XP docking is performed to get ligand: receptor complexes (http://www.schrodinger.com).

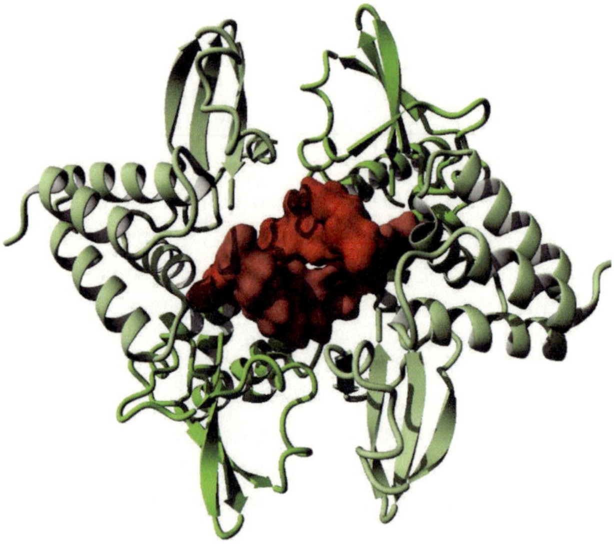

Figure 5. Interaction of VP35 tetramer with dsRNA. The picture shows how VP35 sequestrates dsRNA, which is vital for immunoresponse at cellular level.

3.3. VP24 is vital for budding and acts also as interferon antagonist

VP24 is a secondary matrix protein that is colocalized with VP40 in virions and it is important for intracellular nucleocapsid assembly. It is also a type I interferon antagonist. This protein plays an important role in the budding. VP24 by itself has features that are common to the viral matrix protein (VP40), such as hydrophobicity, membrane binding, and self-oligomerisation [26]. An important role of VP24 in the process of nucleocapsid formation has been demonstrated using electron microscopy [27].

Secondary matrix protein VP24 is one of the virion proteins that play a crucial role in Ebola virus disease pathology [28]. Recently, VP24 was recognized as a major virulent factor. The virulent action of VP24 is initiated by binding of interferon (IFN) to the IFN receptors located on the host cells' surface. The activation of interferon leads to activation of STAT1 protein via Janus tyrosine kinase (JAK1). Activated by phosphorylation, STAT1 forms a dimer that subsequently interacts with KPNA5 (karyopherin 5, also known as importin). KPNA5 is vital for translocation of STAT1 dimer into the nucleus where STAT1 acts as a transcription activator for the expression of IFN stimulated genes. Recent studies have also shown that VP24 competes with STAT1 to bind KPNA5. These studies have shown that KPNA5 binds to VP24 more than 100 times tighter than to the STAT1:STAT1 dimer [29]. The sequestration of free KPNA5 finally results in prevention of STAT1:STAT1 entrance into the nucleus and blocks the subsequent activation of numerous genes that are involved in antiviral activity. The mechanism of VP24 interferon signal path inhibitory action is shown in **Figure 6**.

Garcia-Dorival *et al.* have elucidated VP24's interactome to get better overview of protein functionality. Using label-free quantitative proteomics, they confirmed several known interactions between VP24 and cell proteins and discovered some new ones. They highlighted the interaction between VP24 and integral membrane protein ATP1A1, which is involved in osmoregulation and cell signaling. The researchers have deduced activity of EBOV by disruption of the interaction between ATP1A1 and VP24 with small molecule inhibitor. ATP1A1 could be a promising target for structure-based design of cure against EVD [30].

Another successful approach of protection against EBOV infection is to use phosphorodiamidate morpholino oligomers (PMOs), which are able to bind mRNA in a sequence-specific fashion. The study of Warren *et al.* revealed that PMOs targeting VP24 alone was sufficient to protect Rhesus monkey from lethal infection, while targeting VP35 alone resulted in no protection. The outcome of the study was to confirm VP24 as a key factor for virulence, and additionally, the researchers highlighted PMOs as promising therapeutics against EBOV infection [31].

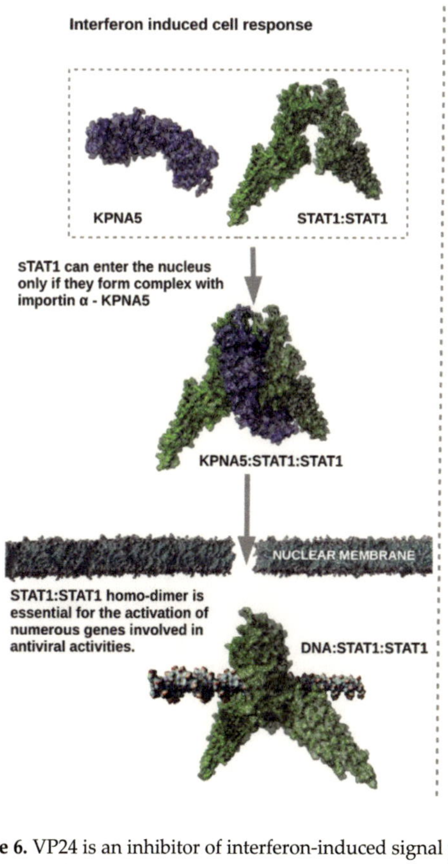

Figure 6. VP24 is an inhibitor of interferon-induced signal path. Normal interferon-induced cell response that results in expression of numerous genes involved in antiviral activity (left), while interferon-induced cell response in the presence of EBOV VP24 is presented on the right side.

Molecules that bind to the VP24 surface where KPNA5 interacts could be inhibitors of viral action of VP24. Pleško *et al.* suggested some compounds from Mediterranean plants as possible inhibitors of interaction between VP24 and KPNA5 [23]. Some of these compounds are listed in **Figure 7**.

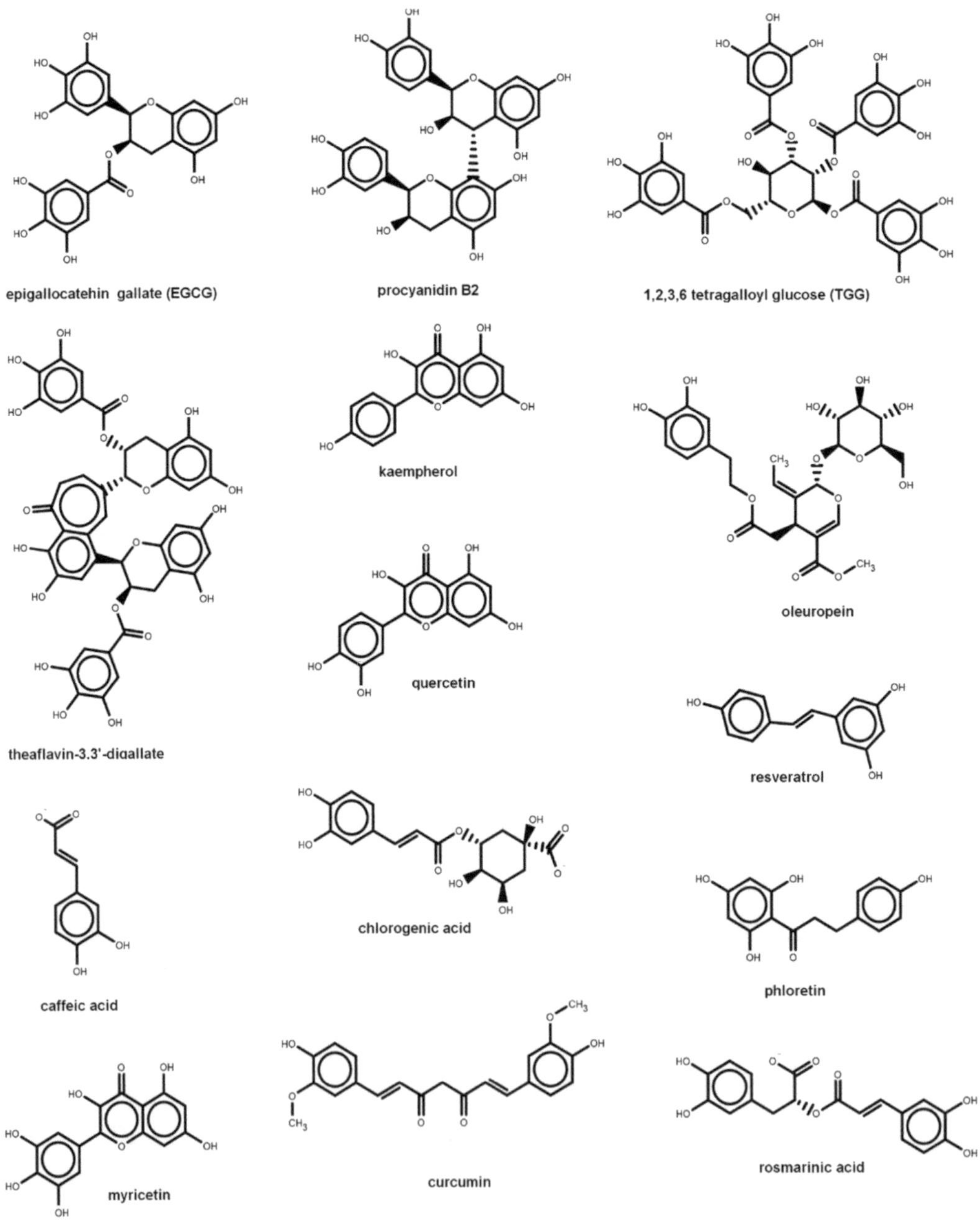

Figure 7. The collection of natural compounds selected for *in silico* search for inhibitors of the interaction between KPNA5 and Ebola's VP24 [23].

This study by Pleško *et al.* has shown that several plant polyphenols, such as epigallocatechin gallate (EGCG), 1,2,3,6-tetragalloyl glucose, theaflavin-3,3'-digallate, and oleuropein, have relevant *in silico* affinity to VP24 [23]. *In silico* studies of Kasmi *et al.* have also indicated that oleuropein, an active ingredient of olive leafs, can interact with EBOV's proteins VP24 and VP30 [32]. Poses of EGCG and oleuropein within binding site of VP24 are shown in **Figure 8**.

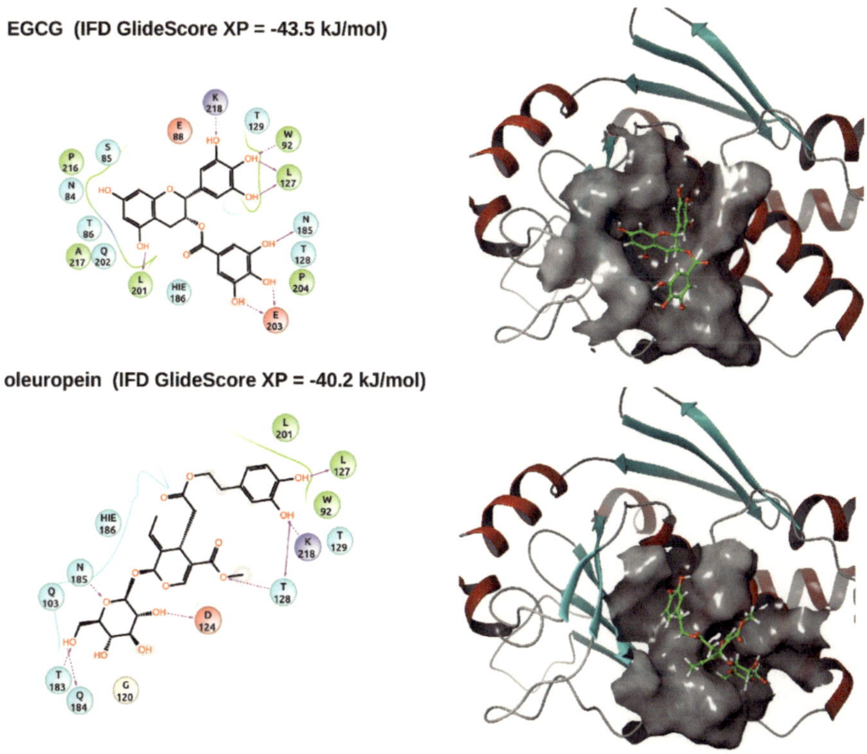

Figure 8. Poses of EGCG and Oleuropein within binding site of VP24. Poses were obtained using Schrodinger's Prime/Glide-Induced Fit Docking protocol [33] (http://www.schrodinger.com).

3.4. Secondary nucleoprotein VP30

The Ebola protein VP30 is known as a secondary nucleoprotein, the protein is colocalized with the nucleoprotein (NP) in inclusion bodies when both proteins are coexpressed *in vitro*. It is evident, from a crystal structure, that the VP30 C-terminal domain is responsible for the interaction with the NP [34]. It has been also shown that VP30 acts as a transcriptional activator only in oligomeric form [35], while binding to the NP oligomerization of VP30 is not required. *In vitro* experiments have shown that the N-terminal domain of the protein is involved in interaction with filoviruses' single-stranded RNAs. Mutagenesis studies have demonstrated Glu197, Arg179, Lys180, and Lys183 in VP30 as key residues essential for nucleocapsid association and transcription activation [8]. The Lys180 centered binding site may be appropriate as a target for small molecules that will act as inhibitors of transcriptional activation and thus behave as effective antiviral agents. The structure of VP30 in its dimeric form that is responsible for activation of transcriptional process is shown in **Figure 9**.

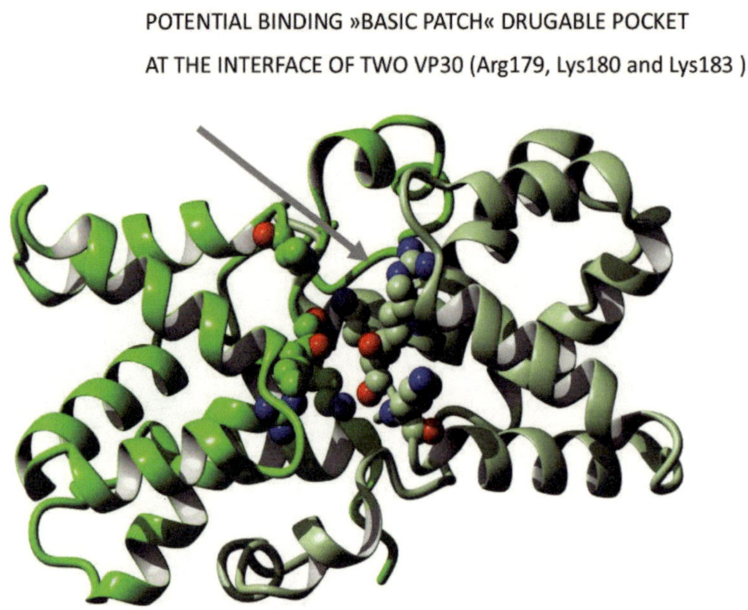

Figure 9. VP30 dimer is required for the activation of transcriptional activity.

The study of Modrof *et al.* has shown that phosphorylation of VP30 impairs transcription of EVD. Only slightly phosphorylated VP30(6A), processed by replacement of six phosphoserines with alanines, is still able to activate EBOV-specific transcription. Mutated VP30 is not able to form inclusion bodies induced by the NP. The authors have also observed that inhibition of intracellular phosphatases with okadaic acid has similar negative impact on the transcriptional activity than replacement of VP30's phosphoserines with aspartate residues. Okadaic acid has no impact on the transcriptional activation by VP30(6A) [36].

3.5. The viral matrix protein VP40

The viral matrix protein VP40 is the most abundant among Ebola virus' proteins, and it is encoded by the most conserved filovirus gene. VP40 is responsible for numerous functions of Ebola virus by rearranging into different oligomeric structures [37]. Each of the structure has different role in the EV life cycle. VP40 dimer traffics to the cellular membrane, where the electrostatic interactions induce its rearrangement into a linear hexamer. VP40 hexamers form a multilayered matrix filament that is critical for budding of virion. Another structural rearrangement of VP40 is in the form of an octameric ring. The RNA-binding VP40 octameric ring is important for the regulation of viral transcription [38]. Different assemblies of VP40 are shown in **Figure 10**.

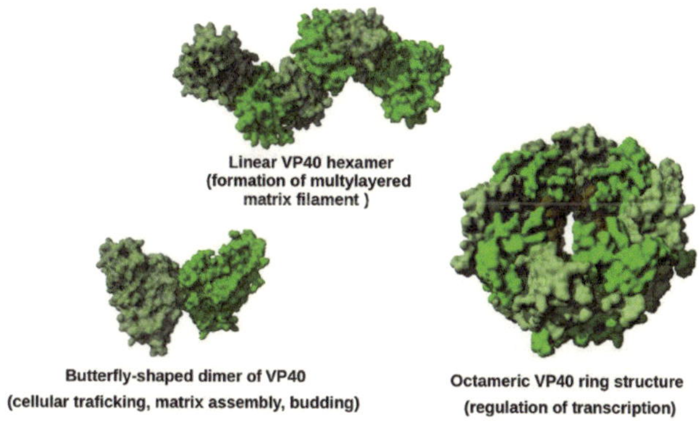

Figure 10. Different assembly of VP40 is required for its distinct functions [39].

The VP40 dimer with some of the potential sites for inhibition of viral budding is shown in **Figure 11** [39]. The area inside the magenta sphere represents the N-terminal domain interface that is responsible for the dimer formation. This interface domain involves two alpha helices 52-65 and 108-117, it is mainly composed of hydrophobic residues, thus the hydrophobic effect could be the driving force in the dimerization. It has been shown that mutation of Leu 117 disrupts the formation of VP40 dimers and inhibits viral budding. The C-terminal domain hexameric interface is shown in red. Met 241 and Ile 307 are residues that are mainly involved in the formation of hexamers. Disruption of the hexameric domain by a set of mutations reduces viral budding from plasma membranes. The cationic patch (blue area) consists of numerous positively charged residues: Lys 224, Lys 225, Lys 274, and Lys 275, which may interact via electrostatic interactions with the anionic leaflet of the plasma membrane. Mutation of these Lys residues reduces the viral budding. The area within the green sphere represents a hydrophobic loop, which penetrates into the plasma membrane—this step is necessary for viral budding.

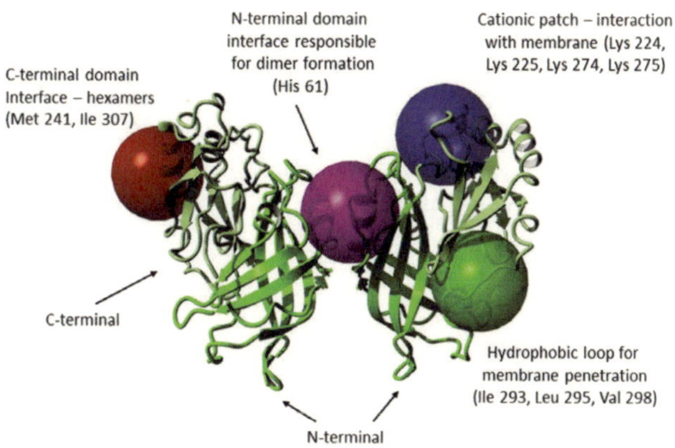

Figure 11. Potential binding sites of small molecules to block viral budding activity of VP40 dimer.

3.6. Ebola virus surface's glycoprotein

The EBOV glycoprotein decorates the surface of virions, and it is responsible for the attachment of virus to the receptor cells and subsequent entry into the cells. Glycoprotein ($GP_{1,2}$) is a transmembrane protein composed of two subunits, GP_1 and GP_2, linked by a disulfide bond. N- and O-linked glycosylation accounts for about one-third of the molecular mass [40]. The posttranslational cleavage of the precursor GP into GP_1 (~160 kDa) and GP_2 (~38-45 kDa) is required for successful infection. Both subunits have an important role in the mechanism of viral infection: heavily glycosylated GP_1 is responsible for the attachment to host cells, while GP_2 is responsible for fusion of the viral and host-cell membrane once the virion has entered the endosome (lysosome). Both subunits have functional domains that are reported to have activities not connected with binding and entry. GP_1, for example, has a domain at the N-terminus, which suppresses lymphocyte blastogenesis *in vitro*. Released GP_1 also has a mucin-like domain (MLD) decorated with glycans. Its function is to prevent neutralizing antibodies from binding to $GP_{1,2}$ at the viral surface. GP_2 has N-terminal motif that exerts immunosuppressive activity. A variety of host cell factors have been connected with EBOV binding and entry: DC-SIGN, L-SIGN, B-integrins, folate receptor A, etc. [41, 42]. Once the virion is inside the endosome, endosomal proteases, mainly cathepsin B, are required for removal of the GP_1 subunit from GP_2. The interaction between NPC-1 and GP_2 has been identified as vital for fusion of the viral and cellular membrane. The role of NPC-1 in EBOV life cycle and the possibilty to use NPC1 as a valuable target for the inhibition of EBOV's escape from the late endosome will be described in a separate subchapter.

An innovative approach to prevent adhesion of EBOV to host cell is blocking receptors (DC-SIGN, L-SIGN) located at the cell surface with glycodendritic structures. DC-SIGN (dendritic cell specific intercellular adhesion molecule-3-grabbing non-integrin) is one of the most important pathogen recognition receptors [43]. This lectin is specific for the recognition of highly mannosylated branched oligosaccharides of EBOV's glycoprotein. Since the affinity between the single copy of the oligosaccharide and its respective receptor is often weak, researchers used the approach of multivalency to enhance the activity. Researchers have developed a series of dendritic glycoconjugates such as Boltorn-type glycodendrimers, glycodendrofullerenes, and virus-like gycodendronanoparticles [44–46]. Some representatives

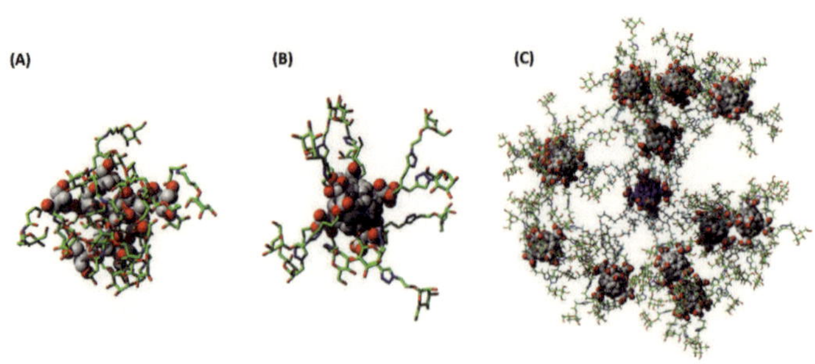

Figure 12. Dendrimeric glycoconjugates: (A) Boltorn-type (16 copies of mannose); (B) glycodendrofullerene (12 copies of mannose); (C) tridecafullerene's superstructure decorated with 120 copies of mannose.

http://dx.doi.org/10.5772/63502

of dendrimeric structures that could successfully bind to the receptors at the host cell surface with high affinity are depicted in **Figure 12**.

In the most recent approach, researchers have synthesized globular multivalent glycofullerenes that act as potent inhibitors in a model of EBOV infection [11]. They recognize hexakis adducts of 60-fullerene as useful building blocks since the obtained products maintain globular shape and with the aspect that it is relatively easy to control the size and multivalency.

Targeting GPs exposed at the surface of EBOV with neutralizing antibodies is one of the most often used strategies in the fight against Ebola. The GP structure represented in **Figure 13** includes neutralizing antibodies from a person who survived infection by the virus. The antibodies bind to the bottom side of the glycoprotein, the portion of protein essential for the process of fusion, which is not usually decorated by oligosaccharidic chains.

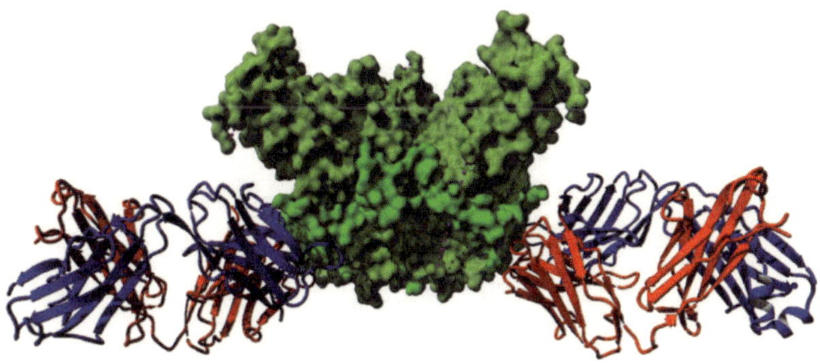

Figure 13. Interaction of glycoprotein with a monoclonal antibody from survived patient (PDB-ID:3csv).

3.7. The human Niemann-Pick disease type C1 protein

The human Niemann-Pick disease type C1 (NPC1) is a membrane protein that is predominantly required for intracellular transport of cholesterol and lipids in mammals. A deficiency of this protein leads to abnormal accumulation of lipids and cholesterol within cells. Recent studies of Côté *et al.* indicated NPC1 protein as an important step for cellular entry of Ebola virus and some other filoviruses [47]. The authors have shown that cultured cells with mutant NPC1 are more resistant to infection with Ebola or Marburg (MARV) filovirus than wild-type cells. Another important finding was that cells treated with imipramine, a tricyclic antidepressant that causes a cellular phenotype similar to NPC1 deficiency, are also more resistant to the infection with EBOV and MARV than untreated cells. In mouse models of EBOV and MARV infection, the animals with deficiency of NPC1 had significantly greater survival ratio than wild type mice. Cunnigham *et al.* screened a small library of compounds and showed that a small molecule inhibitor based on benzylpiperazine-adamantane scaffold almost completely inhibits EBOV infection by blocking interaction between human NPC1 and viral GP_2 [47].

The proposed model for Ebola virus entry via binding of Ebola virus to NPC1 is presented in **Figure 14**. Binding of EBOV to the receptors (DC-SIGN [48, 49], TIM-1 [50], …) at the cell surface is the first and essential step in the viral infection. After successful attachment, the viruses undergo endocytosis and enter the cell internalized in late endosomes. In the next phase, cysteine proteases, primarily cathepsin B, cleave EBOV-GP to a 19-kD fragment. The cleaved EBOV-GP serves as a ligand for NPC1, a multimembrane spanning cholesterol transport protein. After binding of EBOV-GP to NPC1, EBOV nucleocapsid is released into the cell cytosol.

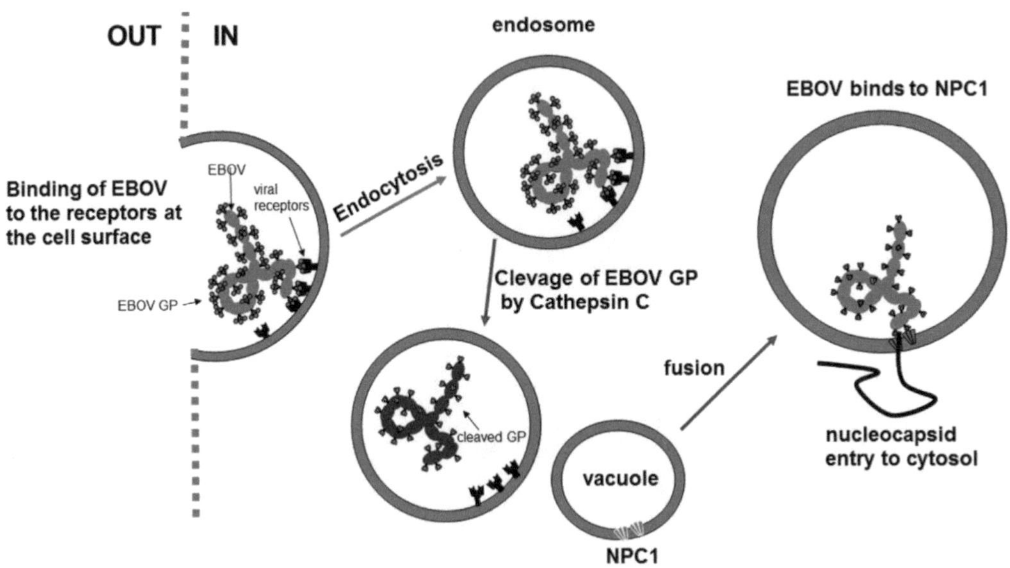

Figure 14. In the first phase, EBOV-GP mediates viral attachment to the cell membrane, which is followed by endocytosis. The glycoproteins that cover the surface of EBOV are cleaved by cathepsin B protease that removes highly glycosylated domains (GP1) to expose the putative receptor-binding domain (GP2) of the glycoprotein. In the next phase, the vacuole that contains NPC1 protein and endosome containing virus fuse together. The virus binds to NPC1 and then is released into the cytoplasm.

We are expecting further development of antivirals for blocking endosomal escape since the structure of the EBOV's GP_2 to its endosomal receptor Niemann-Pick C1 has been recently solved [51].

4. Recent status of EBOV drugs

The most recent outbreak of Ebola viral disease in West Africa 2014 initiated a worldwide activity of searching for an effective cure against one of the most threatening diseases. Numerous bio/med/pharm researches are devoted to the investigation of the action of EBOV at the molecular level as a way to find optimal strategies to combat the virus. In this section, we will describe some small molecule inhibitors that have proven *in vitro* or *in vivo* activity against EBOV infection. In this section, we have followed compound classifications proposed by Picazo *et al.* [52], which is based on their reported mechanism of action (e.g. inhibition of viral replication) and/or documented molecular mechanism (e.g. kinase inhibitors). This section summarizes the identification of numerous compounds with a promising anti-Ebola activity. The reader could find more detailed information related to EBOV small molecule inhibitors in the review articles of Shurtleff *et al.* [11] and others [52–57].

4.1. Viral transcription modulators

An example of small molecules that alter the process of transcription of EBOV's genome is favipiravir (**Figure 15**), which was developed as a selective inhibitor of influenza virus replication (inhibits the viral RNA-dependent RNA polymerase). The antiviral potential against EBOV of favipiravir has been recently tested in a small animal model. Total prevention of mortality of the small animals subjected to the EBOV infection was achieved in these experiments [14]. The nucleoside analog BCX4430 (**Figure 15**) is another compound from the class of viral transcription modulators. BCX4430 is active in vitro against negative-sense RNA-viruses including EBOV. Laboratory tests of BCX4430's anti-EBOV activity have shown a survival rate between 90% and 100 % of experimentally infected mice. Further experiments reported success with a protective action of BCX4430 in EBOV infection of non human primates [58]. C-c3Ado and c3Nep, which were first reported as S-adenosylhomocysteine hydrolase (SAH) inhibitors, are additional examples of compounds with protective action against small animal experimental EBOV infection [59].

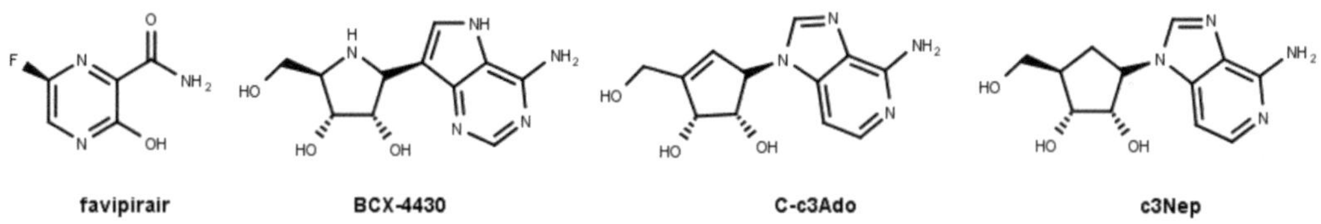

Figure 15. Representative compounds that modulate viral transcription with reported anti-Ebola viral activity.

4.2. Viral entry and fusion modulators

The fusion of EBOV and host cell membrane represents the first phase of EBOV infection [60]. It has been shown that proteolysis of EBOV's glycoprotein $GP_{1,2}$ represents an obligatory step in virus' life cycle. Proteolytic degradation of $GP_{1,2}$ was successfully blocked using inhibitors of cysteine proteases, among which E-64d (unselective protease inhibitor), CA-074 (selective cathepsin B inhibitor), FY-DMK (Cathepsin B/L inhibitor) and Z-FY-(t-Bu)-DMK (Cathepsin L inhibitor), which are shown in **Figure 16** [60, 61]. It was shown that Leupeptin (inhibitor of serine protease) and CIS23631927 – Cat L inhibitor were able to reduce EBOV infection in macrophages and human embryonic cells [62].

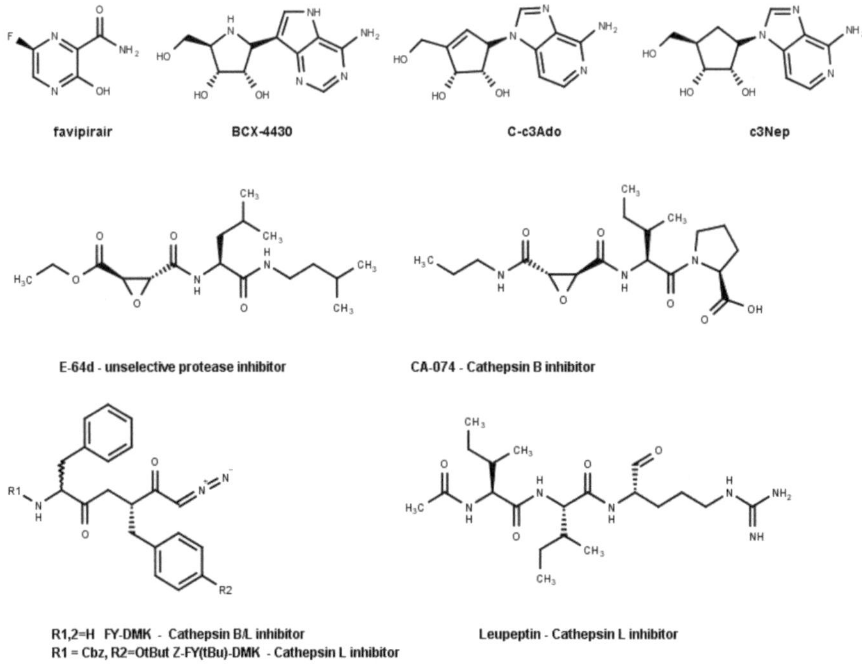

Figure 16. Protease inhibitors with anti-Ebola activity.

Basu *et al.* reported that compounds based on benzodiazepinic scaffold could be used as inhibitors of EBOV entry process. The authors hypothesized that benzodiazepines interfere with proteases by binding to a hydrophobic pocket of the EBOV GP_1-GP_2 interface. A representative benzodiazepine is shown at **Figure 17** [63].

After fusion, the entry of viral particles is followed by endocytosis, which is dependent on a functional cytoskeleton. The research of Yonezawa *et al.* showed the importance of microtubule stabilisation in the process of viral entry. They observed enhanced virus entry in the presence of microtubule stabilizer taxol, on the other hand microtubules' destabilization using nocodazole and colchicine significantly impaired entry process [64].

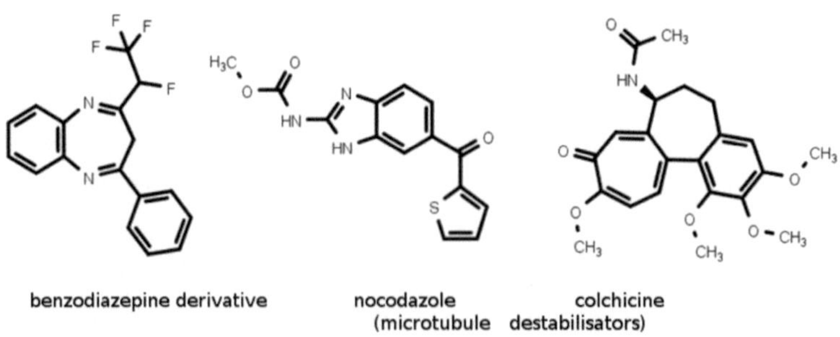

Figure 17. The benzodiazepine derivatives hinder proteases and two microtubules' destabilization.

After fusion with the membrane and subsequent macropinocytosis, the Ebola virus is catched in late endosomes. Carette *et al.* indicated that Niemann-Pick C1 (cholesterol transporter) protein assists in virus escape from endosome to host cell's cytosol [65]. They also showed that impairment of NPC1 (NPC1 phenotype) function of the cell by genetic manipulation leads to complete resistance to EBOV infection. Further research showed that resistance to EBOV infection could be achieved also with U18666A and imipramine, two agents that are known to induce the NPC1 phenotype. In line with these researches, Cote *et al.* indicated piperazine derivative 3.47 as an effective inhibitor of cellular entry by viruses pseudotyped with EBOV-$GP_{1,2}$ [47]. Screen of database of FDA-approved drugs revealed that clomiphene and toremifene (estrogen receptor modulators) strongly inhibited EBOV infection *in vitro*. The action of these two compounds is resulted in accumulation of cholesterol in endosomes, which is typical for impaired NPC1 [66]. The most representatives of NPC-1 inhibitors are shown in **Figure 18**.

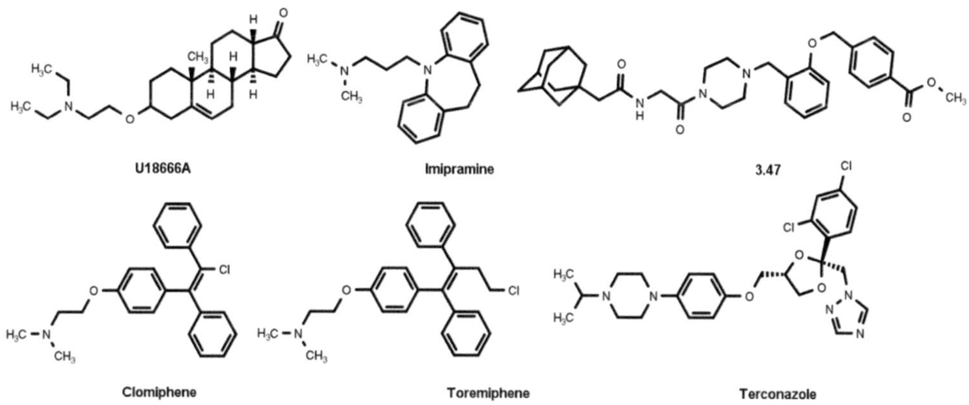

Figure 18. NPC-1 inhibitors are useful as medicaments against EBOV infection.

EBOV-GP, as the key recognition element, represents a crucial mediator of viral budding; therefore, suppression of protein glycosylation is another option to decrease EBOV infection. An example of such treatment is the use of tunicamycin, a N-glycosylation suppressor, which decreases EBOV infection of HeLa cells by more than 90%. Another way to reduce EBOV infectivity is to use imino sugars (IHVR11029, IHVR17028, and IHVR19029) as inhibitors of -glucosidase I, a glycosyl hydrolase from endoplasmic reticulum, which is responsible for proper folding and maturation of nascent proteins [67].

4.3. Signal pathway modulators

Perturbation of cell signaling pathways involved in EBOV infection is another option to inhibit the devastating action of the virus. Here we will describe a few examples where existing kinase and protease inhibitors were used as a cure for EVD.

siRNA screening of human kinome identified mitogen-activated kinase (MAPK), phosphoinositide 3 kinase (PI3K) [68], and calcium/calmodulin kinases (CAMK2) as novel cellular targets for therapeutic intervention against EBOV infection [69]. Garcia *et al.* have shown that c-Abl1 tyrosine kinase is involved in phosphorylation and activation of VP40, the viral protein required for the transport of the viral genome-protein complex to the cell surface and subsequent budding. They reported that inhibition of c-Abl1 kinase with nilotinib and imatinib significantly reduce EBOV replication *in vitro* [70].

By contrast, only dephosphorylated form of VP30, part of EBOV nucleocapsid complex, is required for viral transcription. Studies of Modrof *et al.* exposed that okadaic acid, inhibitor of protein phosphatases 1 (PP1) and 2A (PP2A), both responsible for VP30 dephosphorylation, significantly blocked EBOV growth *in vitro* [36].

The use of ion channel blockers was also used to affect the complex process of viral entry, an example of such approach is to use multiple ion channel blockers amiodarone, dronedarone, and the calcium channel blocker verapamil for inhibition of Ebola virus $GP_{1,2}$-mediated cell entry [71].

Structures of representative signal pathway modulators are presented in **Figure 19**.

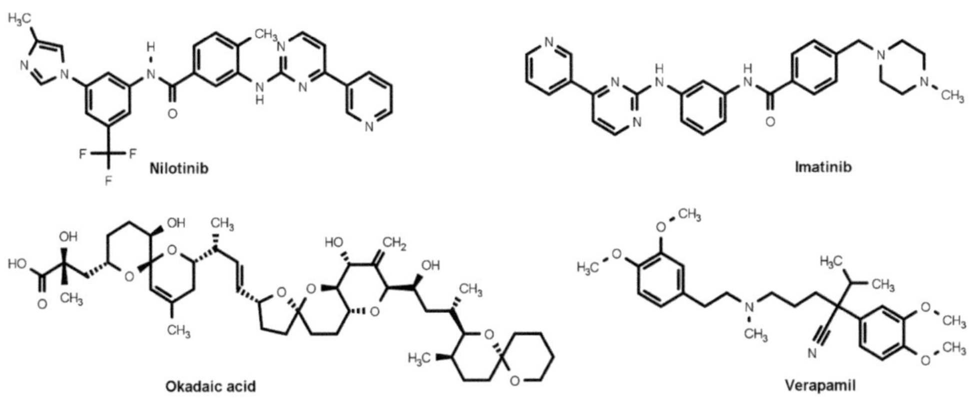

Figure 19. Structures of signal pathway modulators.

4.4. Small molecule Ebola virus modulators *in vitro* and *in vivo*

The review of Picazo *et al.* has collected several different chemotypes, which were shown to impair EVD infection *in vitro* [52]. The collection of structurally diverse compounds, targeting different proteins that are related to pathology of EVD, is shown in **Figure 20**. This collection contains: compound 17-AAG, which represents a heat shock protein 90 (HSP90) inhibitor; ouabain the ATP1A1 (sodium/potassium-transporting ATPase subunit alpha-1) inhibitor, which probably affects the function of VP24; glycyrrhizic acid that acts as the 11beta-hydroxysteroid dehydrogenase inhibitor; bafilomycin A1 and concanamycin A the inhibitors of V-ATPase; and retinazone, which disrupts EBOV infection via binding to glucocorticoid receptor (**Figure 20**).

Representatives of *in vivo* inhibitors are FGI-104 (derivate of amodiaquine, an antimalarial drug) and chloroquine (**Figure 20**). FGI-104 has a broad-spectrum of antiviral activities *in*

http://dx.doi.org/10.5772/63502

vitro, including EBOV, Hepatitis virus B and C, and Cowpox virus among others. The *in vivo* study of experimental Ebola infection of mice has shown excellent prophylactic action of FGI-104. A 10 mg/kg dose of FGI-104 (2 hours before infection) yielded 100% survival [72]. Nowadays, chloroquine is one of the best *in vitro* EBOV inhibitors. Moreover, *in vivo* studies using chloroquine against EBOV infection have shown a promising surviving potential. This compound was able to reduce mortality by 90% when dosage (90 mg/kg) was given four hours before infection [73].

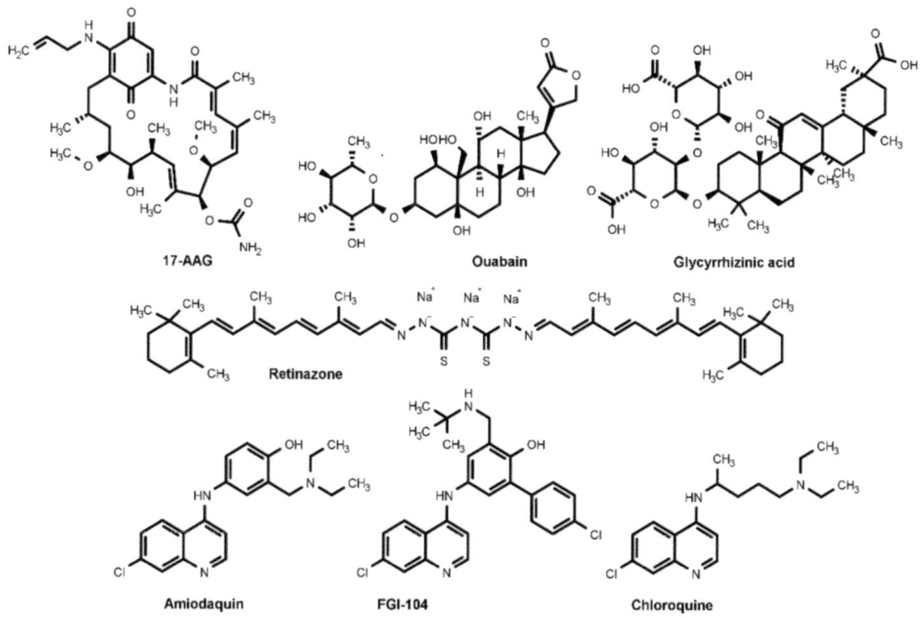

Figure 20. Representatives of *in vitro* and *in vivo* inhibitors of EBOV.

5. Conclusion

Recent outbreak of extremely lethal Ebola hemorrhagic fever in West Africa motivated scientists from all over the world to research EBOV life cycle and the pathology of EVD. The interest to find a successful treatment of Ebola hemorrhagic fever is currently one of the hottest topic in the academy and industry. Our review presents different strategies that could be used for the design of anti-EBOV medications. We have collected what is known about EBOV life cycle, structural information about EBOV protein targets, and some interesting inhibitors in one place. We believe that better knowledge of EBOV life cycle, supported with high quality structural information, could be a deciding factor in accelerating the task of finding a suitable cure against Ebola. Our review has shown that despite a huge collection of data (PDB structures, genome analysis, *in vitro* and in *vivo tests*, etc.) there is still a lot of unknowns about Ebola.

Acknowledgements

This work was supported by Slovenian Research Agency (ARRS) through the research program P1-0201. We are also grateful for the support of dr. Edvard Kobal from Slovenian Science Foundation. And at the end, the authors express their gratitude to Mirzet Čuskić for his continuous moral support of our project.

Author details

Sebastian Pleško and Črtomir Podlipnik*

*Address all correspondence to: crtomir.podlipnik@fkkt.uni-lj.si

Faculty of Chemistry and Chemical Technology, University of Ljubljana, Ljubljana, Slovenia

References

[1] Gire, S.K., et al., *Genomic surveillance elucidates Ebola virus origin and transmission during the 2014 outbreak*. Science, 2014. 345(6202): pp. 1369–72.

[2] Leroy, E.M., et al., *Multiple Ebola virus transmission events and rapid decline of central African wildlife*. Science, 2004. 303(5656): pp. 387–90.

[3] Pandey, A., et al., *Strategies for containing Ebola in West Africa*. Science, 2014. 346(6212): pp. 991–5.

[4] Olinger, G.G., Jr., et al., *Delayed treatment of Ebola virus infection with plant-derived monoclonal antibodies provides protection in rhesus macaques*. Proc Natl Acad Sci U S A, 2012. 109(44): pp. 18030–5.

[5] Kreil, T.R., *Treatment of Ebola virus infection with antibodies from reconvalescent donors*. Emerg Infect Dis, 2015. 21(3): pp. 521–3.

[6] Muhlberger, E., *Filovirus replication and transcription*. Future Virol, 2007. 2(2): pp. 205–15.

[7] Weiss, B., G. Davidkova, and L.W. Zhou, *Antisense RNA gene therapy for studying and modulating biological processes*. Cell Mol Life Sci, 1999. 55(3): pp. 334–58.

[8] de La Vega, M.A., et al., *The multiple roles of sGP in Ebola pathogenesis*. Viral Immunol, 2015. 28(1): pp. 3–9.

[9] Wahl-Jensen, V., et al., *Role of Ebola virus secreted glycoproteins and virus-like particles in activation of human macrophages*. J Virol, 2005. 79(4): pp. 2413–9.

[10] Goodsell, D.S., et al., *The RCSB PDB "Molecule of the Month": inspiring a molecular view of biology*. PLoS Biol, 2015. 13(5): p. e1002140.

[11] Shurtleff, A.C., et al., *Therapeutics for filovirus infection: traditional approaches and progress towards in silico drug design*. Expert Opin Drug Discov, 2012. 7(10): pp. 935–54.

[12] Misasi, J., et al., *Structural and molecular basis for Ebola virus neutralization by protective 6 human antibodies*. Science, 2016. 351 (6279):pp. 1343-6.

[13] Nyakatura, E.K., J.C. Frei, and J.R. Lai, *Chemical and structural aspects of Ebola virus entry inhibitors*. ACS Infect Dis, 2015. 1(1): pp. 42–52.

[14] Furuta, Y., et al., *In vitro and in vivo activities of anti-influenza virus compound T-705*. Antimicrob Agents Chemother, 2002. 46(4): pp. 977–81.

[15] Dong, S., et al., *Insight into the Ebola virus nucleocapsid assembly mechanism: crystal structure of Ebola virus nucleoprotein core domain at 1.8 A resolution*. Protein Cell, 2015. 6(5): pp. 351–62.

[16] Binning, J.M., et al., *Development of RNA aptamers targeting Ebola virus VP35*. Biochemistry, 2013. 52(47): pp. 8406–19.

[17] Noda, T., et al., *The importance of the NP: VP35 ratio in Ebola virus nucleocapsid formation*. J Infect Dis, 2011. 204(Suppl. 3): pp. S878–83.

[18] Kirchdoerfer, R.N., et al., *Assembly of the Ebola virus nucleoprotein from a chaperoned VP35 complex*. Cell Rep, 2015. 12(1): pp. 140–9.

[19] Basler, C.F., et al., *The Ebola virus VP35 protein functions as a type I IFN antagonist*. Proc Natl Acad Sci U S A, 2000. 97(22): pp. 12289–94.

[20] Brown, C.S., et al., *In silico derived small molecules bind the filovirus VP35 protein and inhibit its polymerase cofactor activity*. J Mol Biol, 2014. 426(10): pp. 2045–58.

[21] Prins, K.C., et al., *Basic residues within the ebolavirus VP35 protein are required for its viral polymerase cofactor function*. J Virol, 2010. 84(20): pp. 10581–91.

[22] Dapiaggi, F., S. Pieraccini, and M. Sironi, *In silico study of VP35 inhibitors: from computational alanine scanning to essential dynamics*. Mol Biosyst, 2015. 11(8): pp. 2152–7.

[23] Plesko, S., et al., *In silico study of plant polyphenols' interactions with VP24-Ebola virus membrane-associated protein*. Acta Chim Slov, 2015. 62(3): pp. 555–64.

[24] Leung, D.W., et al., *Structural basis for dsRNA recognition and interferon antagonism by Ebola VP35*. Nat Struct Mol Biol, 2010. 17(2): pp. 165–72.

[25] Mitchell, W.M. and W.A. Carter, *The quest for effective Ebola treatment: Ebola VP35 is an evidence-based target for dsRNA drugs*. Emerg Microbes Infect, 2014. 3(10): p. e77.

[26] Han, Z., et al., *Biochemical and functional characterization of the Ebola virus VP24 protein: implications for a role in virus assembly and budding*. J Virol, 2003. 77(3): pp. 1793–800.

[27] Noda, T., et al., *Regions in Ebola virus VP24 that are important for nucleocapsid formation.* J Infect Dis, 2007. 196(Suppl. 2): pp. S247–50.

[28] Mateo, M., et al., *VP24 is a molecular determinant of Ebola virus virulence in guinea pigs.* J Infect Dis, 2011. 204(Suppl. 3): pp. S1011–20.

[29] Xu, W., et al., *Ebola virus VP24 targets a unique NLS binding site on karyopherin alpha 5 to selectively compete with nuclear import of phosphorylated STAT1.* Cell Host Microbe, 2014. 16(2): pp. 187-200.

[30] Garcia-Dorival, I., et al., *Elucidation of the Ebola virus VP24 cellular interactome and disruption of virus biology through targeted inhibition of host-cell protein function.* J Proteome Res, 2014. 13(11): pp. 5120–35.

[31] Warren, T.K., et al., *A single phosphorodiamidate morpholino oligomer targeting VP24 12 protects rhesus monkeys against lethal Ebola virus infection.* MBio, 2015. 6(1):pp. e02344-14.

[32] Kasmi, Y., *In silico study of the inhibitory effects of oleuropein, kaempferol, and quercetin on the VP30 protein from ebola virus.* Int J Innov Appl Stud, 2014. 8(4): pp. 1566–73.

[33] Sherman, W., et al., *Novel procedure for modeling ligand/receptor induced fit effects.* J Med Chem, 2006. 49(2): pp. 534–53.

[34] Hartlieb, B., et al., *Crystal structure of the C-terminal domain of Ebola virus VP30 reveals a role in transcription and nucleocapsid association.* Proc Natl Acad Sci U S A, 2007. 104(2): pp. 624–9.

[35] Hartlieb, B., et al., *Oligomerization of Ebola virus VP30 is essential for viral transcription and can be inhibited by a synthetic peptide.* J Biol Chem, 2003. 278(43): pp. 41830–6.

[36] Modrof, J., et al., *Phosphorylation of VP30 impairs Ebola virus transcription.* J Biol Chem, 2002. 277(36): pp. 33099–104.

[37] Bornholdt, Z.A., et al., *Structural rearrangement of ebola virus VP40 begets multiple functions in the virus life cycle.* Cell, 2013. 154(4): pp. 763–74.

[38] Hoenen, T., et al., *VP40 octamers are essential for Ebola virus replication.* J Virol, 2005. 79(3): pp. 1898–905.

[39] Stahelin, R.V., *Could the Ebola virus matrix protein VP40 be a drug target?* Expert Opin Ther Targets, 2014. 18(2): pp. 115–20.

[40] Volchkov, V.E., *Processing of the Ebola virus glycoprotein.* Curr Top Microbiol Immunol, 1999. 235: pp. 35–47.

[41] Alvarez, C.P., et al., *C-type lectins DC-SIGN and L-SIGN mediate cellular entry by Ebola virus in cis and in trans.* J Virol, 2002. 76(13): pp. 6841–4.

[42] Marzi, A., et al., *Analysis of the interaction of Ebola virus glycoprotein with DC-SIGN (dendritic cell-specific intercellular adhesion molecule 3-grabbing nonintegrin) and its homologue DC-SIGNR.* J Infect Dis, 2007. 196(Suppl. 2): pp. S237–46.

[43] Geijtenbeek, T.B., A. Engering, and Y. Van Kooyk, *DC-SIGN, a C-type lectin on dendritic cells that unveils many aspects of dendritic cell biology*. J Leukoc Biol, 2002. 71(6): pp. 921–31.

[44] Luczkowiak, J., et al., *Pseudosaccharide functionalized dendrimers as potent inhibitors of DC-SIGN dependent Ebola pseudotyped viral infection*. Bioconjug Chem, 2011. 22(7): pp. 1354–65.

[45] Muñoz, A., et al., *Synthesis of giant globular multivalent glycofullerenes as potent inhibitors in a model of Ebola virus infection*. Nat Chem, 2016. 8(1): pp. 50–7.

[46] Rojo, J. and R. Delgado, *Glycodendritic structures: promising new antiviral drugs*. J Antimicrob Chemother, 2004. 54(3): pp. 579–81.

[47] Cote, M., et al., *Small molecule inhibitors reveal Niemann-Pick C1 is essential for Ebola virus infection*. Nature, 2011. 477(7364): pp. 344–8.

[48] Lasala, F., et al., *Mannosyl glycodendritic structure inhibits DC-SIGN-mediated Ebola virus infection in cis and in trans*. Antimicrob Agents Chemother, 2003. 47(12): pp. 3970–2.

[49] Baribaud, F., R.W. Doms, and S. Pohlmann, *The role of DC-SIGN and DC-SIGNR in HIV and Ebola virus infection: can potential therapeutics block virus transmission and dissemination?* Expert Opin Ther Targets, 2002. 6(4): pp. 423–31.

[50] Kondratowicz, A.S., et al., *T-cell immunoglobulin and mucin domain 1 (TIM-1) is a receptor for Zaire Ebolavirus and Lake Victoria Marburgvirus*. Proc Nat Acad Sci, 2011. 108(20): pp. 8426–31.

[51] Wang, H., et al., *Ebola viral glycoprotein bound to its endosomal receptor Niemann-Pick C1*. Cell, 2016. 164(1): pp. 258–68.

[52] Picazo, E. and F. Giordanetto, *Small molecule inhibitors of ebola virus infection*. Drug Discov Today, 2015. 20(2): pp. 277–86.

[53] Izawa, K., et al., *Small-molecule therapeutics for ebola virus (EBOV) disease treatment*. Eur J Organ Chem, 2016. 2016(1): pp. 8–16.

[54] Janeba, Z., *Development of small-molecule antivirals for Ebola*. Med Res Rev, 2015. 35(6): pp. 1175–94.

[55] Litterman, N., C. Lipinski, and S. Ekins, *Small molecules with antiviral activity against the Ebola virus*. F1000Res, 2015. 4: p. 38.

[56] Mendoza, E.J., X. Qiu, and G.P. Kobinger, *Progression of Ebola therapeutics during the 2014–2015 outbreak*. Trends Mol Med, 2016. 22(2): pp. 164–173.

[57] Wu, C.R.-Y.Z., *Small molecule inhibitors against Ebola virus: research advances*. JIPR, 2015. 42(1): pp. 49–61.

[58] Warren, T.K., et al., *Protection against filovirus diseases by a novel broad-spectrum nucleoside analogue BCX4430*. Nature, 2014. 508(7496): pp. 402–5.

[59] Huggins, J., Z.X. Zhang, and M. Bray, *Antiviral drug therapy of filovirus infections: S-adenosylhomocysteine hydrolase inhibitors inhibit Ebola virus in vitro and in a lethal mouse model*. J Infect Dis, 1999. 179(Suppl. 1): pp. S240–7.

[60] Chandran, K., et al., *Endosomal proteolysis of the Ebola virus glycoprotein is necessary for infection*. Science, 2005. 308(5728): pp. 1643–5.

[61] Schornberg, K., et al., *Role of endosomal cathepsins in entry mediated by the Ebola virus glycoprotein*. J Virol, 2006. 80(8): pp. 4174–8.

[62] Gnirss, K., et al., *Cathepsins B and L activate Ebola but not Marburg virus glycoproteins for efficient entry into cell lines and macrophages independent of TMPRSS2 expression*. Virology, 2012. 424(1): pp. 3–10.

[63] Basu, A., et al., *Identification of a small-molecule entry inhibitor for filoviruses*. J Virol, 2011. 85(7): pp. 3106–19.

[64] Yonezawa, A., M. Cavrois, and W.C. Greene, *Studies of Ebola virus glycoprotein-mediated entry and fusion by using pseudotyped human immunodeficiency virus type 1 virions: involvement of cytoskeletal proteins and enhancement by tumor necrosis factor alpha*. J Virol, 2005. 79(2): pp. 918–26.

[65] Carette, J.E., et al., *Ebola virus entry requires the cholesterol transporter Niemann-Pick C1*. Nature, 2011. 477(7364): pp. 340–3.

[66] Johansen, L.M., et al., *FDA-approved selective estrogen receptor modulators inhibit Ebola virus infection*. Sci Transl Med, 2013. 5(190): p. 190ra79.

[67] Chang, J., et al., *Small molecule inhibitors of ER alpha-glucosidases are active against multiple hemorrhagic fever viruses*. Antiviral Res, 2013. 98(3): pp. 432–40.

[68] Saeed, M.F., et al., *Phosphoinositide-3 kinase-Akt pathway controls cellular entry of Ebola virus*. PLoS Pathog, 2008. 4(8): p. e1000141.

[69] Kolokoltsov, A.A., et al., *Identification of novel cellular targets for therapeutic intervention against Ebola virus infection by siRNA screening*. Drug Dev Res, 2009. 70(4): pp. 255–265.

[70] Garcia, M., et al., *Productive replication of Ebola virus is regulated by the c-Abl1 tyrosine kinase*. Sci Transl Med, 2012. 4(123): p. 123ra24.

[71] Gehring, G., et al., *The clinically approved drugs amiodarone, dronedarone and verapamil inhibit filovirus cell entry*. J Antimicrob Chemother, 2014. 69(8): pp. 2123–31.

[72] Kinch, M.S., et al., *FGI-104: a broad-spectrum small molecule inhibitor of viral infection*. Am J Transl Res, 2009. 1(1): pp. 87–98.

[73] Madrid, P.B., et al., *A systematic screen of FDA-approved drugs for inhibitors of biological threat agents*. PLoS One, 2013. 8(4): p. e60579.